W9-AAX-012

TABLE OF CONTENTS

Fading Angel

A Chronicle of Love

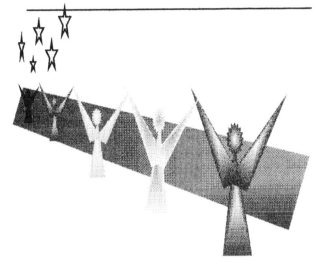

A story of compassion,
understanding and survival amidst
the devastation of

Alzheimer's Disease

Sande Donahue

Fading Angel
A Chronicle of Love

ISBN 0-9706007-0-4

Printed in the U.S.A.

To My Mother

**In tribute
to her courageous journey
into darkness**

Prologue

It is very difficult to know exactly where to begin. The signals are subtle and the denial is ever present. One does not know how or why or when the invasion begins or how it creeps into your life and into the lives of everyone around you. All you know is that something is not right and your worst fears are paraded before you in some sort of taunting, macabre dance. Suddenly, reality grabs hold of you like a boa constrictor, squeezing and squeezing until you can no longer fight. Your only hope for survival is to succumb and face what lies before you, every ugly inch of the path of destruction and deterioration.

When the ever-blessed resolve settles in, you begin to plan for the future. You ponder every option, every opportunity, every alternative. You pray that this is only a joke, a phase or a temporary passage of time. But then, your shoulders slump as you step towards the waiting abyss; you breathe in deeply, take your loved one by the hand, and you both take your plunge into the sea of darkness.

Author's Notes

There are thousands upon thousands of medical books to tell you what to look for. There are support groups all over the country that will aid you in your quest for assistance. There are busloads of people who will give you advice, everyone from your family doctor right down to the local postman. But there is nothing on this planet that can truly prepare you for your loved one's journey through timelessness and spacelessness. There is nothing that gives you the slightest clue of how careful planning and preparation can play a vital role in your own survival as a caregiver. And there is nothing grander than the few moments of spontaneous levity you might experience, even if only fleeting, during this transition from whole to half to zero.

In this book, my own personal diary and chronicle of events, I have attempted to give you some insight into this trauma. It can destroy you, or it can show you that other side of yourself that you have kept hidden so well all these years. That side of you that bleeds compassion and love when you least expect it.

I have attempted to give you ideas on how this journey might be made a little easier not only for yourself, but for that individual who will be suffering from this dreaded disease, this devastating corruption of mind, body and soul referred to as Alzheimer's. I have also included many, many lessons learned along the way, lessons and tips that no one will tell you because no one has the nerve to tell you. Lessons on how to legally circumvent the system, because the system will not tell you. I have included many actual experiences, some horrific, some wonderfully humorous, but all quite possible in your situation, and full of interesting inroads and clues.

In my own mind, I can intellectually understand the scientific explanations of this "cancer-like" erosion that spreads through the brain, eating away at every inch of existence of my Mother's life. But in my heart, I will never understand why such vital, wonderful, intelligent people become stricken with this monster, people like my Mother, who has been my model of living, my mentor, my support, my crutch, *my angel*, who now sits and fades away into nothingness.

I've spent the entire duration of her illness doing whatever I can do to make this journey a little less frightening for her. Because it is, you know. It is probably the most terrifying experience anyone can imagine. But I also know that what I have done and what I continue to do, has made what's left of her life, somewhat bearable.

I continue to strive to create a warm and loving atmosphere, so important for their comfort zone. To be there and be a part of her shattered life whenever she can grasp a tiny moment of reality. To hug . . . and squeeze . . . and kiss her when I see that veil of terror begin to drop. To create laughter when I recognize that glimmer in her eye of long ago.

It's the least I can do . . .

For my Fading Angel.

Chapter 1

The Beginning

"The signals are subtle . . . . . . "

Pie and Coffee

The human brain is a wondrous thing. The human mind is an even more wondrous mystery. Science and medicine have been researching both for centuries and have made tremendous progress in the knowledge and under-standing of their diseases and malfunctions. But because of the extreme complexity of both the mind and the brain, there is so much yet undiscovered and unknown.

It seems that when we contract a physical illness or disease of the body, we step up to the plate and handle it whether it's ours or someone else's.

We feel symptoms, we are diagnosed, we are treated, and we are cured, if we're lucky. We expect answers and cures. If there are no answers, then cures. If there are no cures, then we plan for the future for both ourselves and our loved ones. But when it comes to an "illness" of the brain or the mind, it's freeze up time. No one seems to know how to act or react. With mental dysfunction, everybody hides in the closet. No one plans, no one talks, no one seems to know what to do. We rely on doctors or psychiatrists to tell us what to do. But their job is to diagnose and treat the illness, if they can. Their job is not to tell us how to act or react.

Alzheimer's is a very sneaky and tricky disease that will creep in on you ever so quietly. It is very difficult to detect and to make a determination on whether you have an ensuing problem or simply a natural lessening of abilities due to the natural aging process.

Every individual at one time or another, experiences a forgetfulness or confused state due to stress, too much activity, or too many different focuses. As we age, there is also a natural mental quieting where we will not appear to be as sharp as we once were. One can misplace their keys. Forget to turn off the iron. Leave something at home that we meant to take with us as we walked out the door. Nothing phenomenal, no big deal. However, when extraordinary forgetfulness presents itself repeatedly, a larger than life problem is on the horizon. People tend to overlook these signals, hoping that what may be their worst fear, is not really presenting itself, thereby existing in that dangerous state of denial.

I had just such an experience in 1988 with my Mother. My parents had a summer home in Southern Wisconsin where I religiously trekked off to every week-end. It was a glorious little place in a glorious little town with antique shops, thrift shops, book stores, etc. We would scamper up there as early as possible in the season. Sometimes on an early Spring night, still chilled to the bone by the last threats of winter, we would sit out over a campfire with our winter parkas, drink Old Fashions, and listen to the bullfrogs claim new turf just inches away from us on the water's edge. It was our little Paradise.

One usual week-end, on a Saturday morning, my Mother and I decided to stroll through town and browse the ever-growing line-up of shops. On our way to town, my Mother said, "When we get finished, let's stop for some pie and coffee."

I said, "Great! Sounds like a plan."

We continued on to our first stop, my favorite gift shop. We spent about twenty minutes inside, left to return to the car. Once inside the car, my Mother said, "Hey, honey, when we get finished, let's stop for some pie and coffee."

I didn't pay any attention to the repeated statement and said, "Of course, I told you we would."

We went to the next shop, a little thrift store where my Mother loved to buy the 25 cent novels.

We browsed, returned to the car to continue our adventure. Once inside, my Mother said, "Let's stop for some pie and coffee when we're done."

I momentarily lost control, looked at her and said tersely, "What IS your problem? I told you three times that we would stop for pie and coffee. How many times do I have to say it?" It was one of those moments that you wanted to take back the second it was over and one of those statements where you wanted to cut your tongue off for having spoken it.

To reprieve myself from my dark moment of anger, I said, "You know what? Right now sounds like a great time for some pie and coffee. How about it?"

"Oh, great!" she replied. "Sounds like a good deal."

We went to the little diner, ordered our pie and coffee, and sat for about a half hour talking and visiting with some other folks in the diner. When we finished, we paid the bill, went to the car, and started on our way home. About five minutes down the road, she turned to me and said, "Honey, how would you like to stop for some pie and coffee?"

My heart sank. I knew. This was not a natural forgetfulness or just a tired mind. This was serious business. This was a signal. It was my wake-up call to pay attention and start planning.

When we returned home, my Mother went into the house and I approached my Father and said, "We've got problems." I proceeded to relate the afternoon's events. He replied, "Oh, go on! There's nothing wrong. We do that all the time!" I was amazed at the speed denial had grabbed hold, firmly entwining itself around us as though it had already taken up permanent residency. I knew that its stronghold would be the battle of my life. I needed to begin working on a plan.

Oh brother, did I need a plan.

Chapter 2

"You explore every option . . . . . "

The Plan

Yes, the plan. The biggest plan of your life. The plan that will mean your survival. The plan that will ease the journey for both yourself and your loved one. The plan that will take you from chaos to order and from fear to understanding. We plan for everything from the birth of our first child all the way to our own demise. We plan showers, birthdays, weddings, dinner parties. We buy insurance, we invest in mutual funds, we do everything in our power to *plan* for anything that may come our way. This plan, my friend, will be the one that can make or break you.

Do not take lightly my statements on planning for the future. You may think you have time. You may think that those dreaded *advanced stages* are eons down the road. You may think that "everything will work itself out." Nothing, but nothing, works itself out. You and only you are the King of this Mountain. I cannot emphasize how important it is to plot and plan, discuss, inform, and have all your ducks in line because, believe me, you have no time.

One day it may appear that you have everything under control, and the next day you find yourself drowning in a sea of chaos and confusion. It is so very, very vital to begin working on your plan the very moment you suspect something. Sit down and write yourself an outline. . Here is just a short one to help you get started.

1. Make a list of people of whom you think you might need to discuss your situation. This could include children, your brothers or sisters, brothers and sisters of the victim, parents, grandchildren, nieces, nephews. Anyone in the immediate family that should be aware of the oncoming disease.

2. Make a list of people that you know you are going to need to help and assist you from time to time. This list should include all of the above, but added to it can be your lifelong friends or neighbors, co-workers, anyone that you think would be willing to give you some assistance. Don't be afraid

to discuss anything and especially don't be afraid to ask for help. You will be pleasantly surprised at how many people really do understand and are willing to give a helping hand when you need it.

3. Almost right from the beginning, you will have to think about whether or not the afflicted individual is capable of being left alone or should have someone with them all day. There is always the chance of fire if things are left on the stove, the victim walking out of house and getting lost, any number of problems that you need to be aware of right from the beginning. This will require a daily schedule for you and for others. If you are still working and everyone else you know is working, it may be necessary to go to outside help.

4. See your family doctor immediately and get a certified diagnoses. You will need this for any further activity down the road relative to your preparation.

5. Call an attorney. Make sure your financial matters are in order and make sure wills, house deeds, etc. are signed over to the proper individual who might be the beneficiary of the victim. Also, while the

individual is still in a reasonable state of mind, discuss the matter of a living will and life-sustaining measures. These legal matters will become very, very important later on.

6. Begin making lists of adult day care centers and call each and every one of them for specifics on their care and costs. Get the individual registered immediately.

7. Make a list of organizations or agencies that might provide home care or home help such as housecleaning, meal preparation, or just "baby" sitting services that will give you an opportunity to get out and take care of business or just socialize. If you can depend on family or friends for this, all the better. But be prepared if none of those persons are available.

8. Call the Alzheimer's Association and get your loved one registered with the Safe Return Program. This is a nationwide link that gives the individual a registration number and a bracelet to wear with that registration number and the 800 number for the program. If the victim wanders and gets lost, anyone encountering this person can check the bracelet, call the number,

and the Safe Return program calls you to notify you of the whereabouts of the victim.

9. If the individual is still working, call their employer and have a candid discussion about the disease, their termination, company disability programs, assistance from the company regarding state or federal disability money that might be available to you.

10. Start shopping for waterproof bed sheets and disposable briefs for incontinence. It happens quicker than you might think.

11. And lastly, make preparations for a possible full-time live-in caregiver. I have had a live-in for four years and would have never made it through if I had not had that aid and assistance, not only for my Mother, but for help in the house as well. This can be very, very expensive if you go through the regular agencies. However, sometimes you can find a connection through your church or other persons, or various ethnic organizations who like to bring their relatives here but don't necessarily have the space for them or the money to provide for them. I have used the Polish

newspapers in Chicago and have had extraordinary luck. I have had one woman with me now for almost three of those four years and she has become family. I do not speak Polish, and she doesn't speak English, but between our translation books and our combined efforts to learn key words and phrases in each other's language, we have managed to communicate quite well. We even have a glass of wine together now and then and discuss families, life, news items, etc. And sometimes just have a good laugh. You can get these wonderful angels of mercy relatively inexpensively and they are most grateful for the work. However, you must remember to be kind and generous when need be, holidays, birthdays, etc.

(I will discuss all of the above items at greater length in upcoming chapters with more details and more suggestions.)

As time goes by, you may revise this list as many times as you think you may need to. Remember, this is a roller coaster ride and nothing will go according to plan. But you will find yourself way ahead of the game if you at least start with some kind of an outline. The important thing here is to face head-on whatever it is that may confront you.

My motto is, "Anticipate the unexpected and prepare for the possibilities!"

My purpose here is two-fold. I have tried, in this chapter, to give you a little head start on the more business-like areas of this experience. But this is only the beginning as there will be many obstacles and frustrations in the business arena that you, as the caregiver, are going to encounter. But my other objective here is to give you an insight as to what you can expect in the non-business areas, the areas that you are going to encounter that fall somewhere between mystery and horror, sadness and laughter, pain and delight, every nook and cranny of the unseen, unexpected and uninvited. Having a tiny smidgen of knowledge is going to lighten the load a bit and enlighten you to the doorways, pathways, corridors and tunnels of the journey that your loved one is about to embark. If you're smart, you'll take their hand, and let them know that you're traveling right beside them. Because ultimately, their journey becomes your journey.

To travel this roadway is not easy and certainly is not something that you planned. But as any experience in life has taught you, if you must embark on a different and more difficult endeavor then you had planned on, the best way to do it is with some knowledge and understanding. I started this journey with no knowledge whatsoever and all I had to rely on was my common sense and my determination that whatever was going to happen was not going to get the best of me. Believe me, there were some close calls. But the knowledge I did gain every inch of the way was a blessing. I hope to share this knowledge with you and perhaps make your journey with your loved one a little less bumpy.

Chapter 3

" Something is not right . . . . "

The First Step

I think one of the most important things you can do in the very beginning of this tragic journey is to discuss it openly with your loved one. They need to be made aware that, yes, something *is* wrong. They need to know that <u>you know</u> that something is wrong. That you are concerned and that you are doing everything in your power to make sure that *both* of you are going to be okay through this. They have realized for a long time that something was not right. And they have lived with the confusion for many, many weeks or months, but have not spoken a word. You see, they live with a profound fear. Fear that they will soon be burdening their family and loved ones. Fear that they may be tossed aside or taken away. Fear, every single hour of every single day, that they will be *discovered.*

Society, television, support groups, doctors, panels, workshops, *everyone*, has discussed it openly with families, with caregivers, with spouses. Discussed it with everyone except the *victim.* I think it would be spectacular if someone could start a program of support groups for the Alzheimer's victims! They are the ones who need the support. They are the ones who need to know that they will be cared for, that they are cared for. They are the ones who need to know that they aren't the only ones in the world who have this problem. They are the ones who need to know that they won't be going through this alone, that there is family, friends and outside groups of people who understand and care.

Even though there are medical and scientific explanations of the disease, the terror is so profound even in the beginning stages that *it* alone is probably a factor in the speedy deterioration of the victim. Because terror *can drive you crazy!* People have no problem discussing everything from cancer to Parkinson's to whatever, with the victims of these wretched diseases. But for some reason, there is a taboo about discussing Alzheimer's with the Alzheimer's victim. It's like they won't understand. Believe me, my friends, they understand all too well. And they need to talk about it. They need to know that you are expecting anything and everything and that you will be there no matter what. They need to be told that whatever happens or whatever they do, is *okay with you!* Now remember, every individual is different and I certainly am not a medical doctor, nor am I a psychologist or a psychiatrist. But I strongly believe that most persons who are experiencing this "strangeness", this invasion, will want to know what the hell is going on! My Mother was most grateful to know that I, too, had noticed that "something is not right", and my candid discussions with her eased her anxiety. She was the one who told me about the terror of living with the "strangeness" and the terror of being discovered. She continually asked me if "it was okay", "did I mind", "does it bother me". *"Bother me?!"* I would answer incredulously. "You are my Mother! Nothing, but nothing, you do is going to *bother me! Whatever* you do is okay with me." We would hug and kiss and hold hands. Holding, touching, squeezing, hugging becomes vitally important. This sets the precedent early in their minds and later becomes their signal that you are still there and that everything is still okay. They may forget everything else they've ever known in their entire lives, but they will never forget the feeling of a hug or a kiss or a hand in theirs. My Mother, after fourteen years with this disease, still knows how to pucker up for a kiss.

But to continue on this subject, let me ask a question. If you discovered you had cancer, or were told you had Parkinson's, you would have numerous discussions with doctors, clergy, family and friends regarding your diagnosis, your treatment, your prognosis, your cure, your length of life. Why is it that an Alzheimer's victim is kept completely in the dark? Why are they treated like they are invisible? And why do people talk around them and not *to* them?

How would you feel if you were lying in a hospital bed and you had ten people standing around discussing your terminal illness and never giving you a nod or a wink in regard to it. They would never tell you how you got it, where it came from, what to do about it, what treatment you might have to endure, what pain you might have to endure, and your ultimate demise from it. Now, I certainly am not advocating that you tell an Alzheimer's patient that they are going to die. That just plain isn't a nice thing to do. All terminal illness needs to be discussed with kid gloves, but for heaven's sake, it *does* need to be discussed. But in this case, not clinically. It needs to be discussed compassion-ately and with great care.

The victims need to have it implanted in their minds as they pass through these portals of darkness that love and compassion and hugs and kisses will always be there. That all these things are but an arm's reach away. It is their connection. Perhaps their one and only last connection to a fading reality, blurred by chaotic thoughts, hallucinations and a mindless existence. <u>Be</u> that connection. <u>Be</u> their crutch, their link, their last grasp. If you never discuss it again throughout the duration, make sure you at least have one long and hearty discussion about it with them. Because rest assured, they will be the ones to keep bringing it up, continually seeking the reassurance that you will be there. And that it is okay that "something is not right."

But let's not forgot one very important factor. There are going to be those folks who will be in denial about their loved one having this dreaded disease. But there are also going to be those folks who will be in denial about *having* the disease. In other words, you may begin to approach the subject with your afflicted loved one, and they will totally deny and rebuke any inclination that such a thing exists within them. The best thing to do in this case is to gently continue the conversation and leave the seed planted and let it grow on its own. There will come a day when the victim, him or herself, will have to finally acknowledge that they are, in fact, embarking on this journey. The surrender will be subtle, and you must be gentle in your knowledge of their acceptance.

I have heard of so many cases where the discussion was never brought into play, the afflicted individual continued to live in denial, and the worse the disease became, the more frustrated and violent the victim became. Again, depending on the individual, the issue of violence, in most cases, can be kept to a minimum with a complete understanding of the disease by all.

Bear in mind, that there are some physicians out there who disagree with me on this issue. One physician told me that if you discuss this openly with the patient, you take away all hope and, perhaps, instill more fear than is necessary. And I don't disagree with him. However, as with any terminal illness as in cancer, etc., the patient is always told of their oncoming demise and yet, the idea of taking away their hope or instilling fear is never considered. As the medical industry continues to make strides in all areas of medicine, Alzheimer's is just another area where continued research and inroads to discovery is made every day. And as with any terminal disease, there is always hope that new discoveries will bring relief and/or cures.

I will continue to stress throughout this book that I am not a medical doctor or therapist. I am merely an individual who has lived through this horrific experience and learned, by trial and error, what has worked for me and what didn't. There are many case studies and research that will tell you what you might expect on the violence issue. Again, every individual is different and based on their life experiences, will react accordingly. But with gentle discussion and understanding, things may turn in your favor. As it has been said so many times, the first step is the most difficult, but the most important.

Chapter 4

" The path of destruction . . . ."

Names, Names and More Names

One of the most embarrassing situations in society is meeting someone for the third, fourth or fifth time and forgetting their name each and every time. It would be so much easier if you could simply call them whatever you wanted to or whatever came to your mind first. But, unfortunately, we would be chastised and reprimanded consistently for this kind of behavior. But, you will learn that names, names and more names is one of the first things to disappear from a victim's memory. You may experience many new situations and changes in the habits of the victim. They may lose a purse, or a set of keys, a wallet, maybe even a book or two and perhaps some money. But the names are the real test. Not a test for the victim! Oh no, this is a test for you and everyone else involved with the victim. Sisters become aunts, sons become childhood friends, husbands become brothers, and so on.

My Mother still remembers her sisters, Dorothy and Kelly. Those names are old, old memories. But she has a hard time now even with my name or recognizing me. She does know, of course, that when she sees me she will be getting a huge kiss and a big, big hug. But she can't remember who I am or why I'm giving her those kisses and hugs, but she loves them.

As time goes on, you begin to notice the decades of memory slipping by. The most recent ten years are the first to go, then the next. New people become total strangers. Then friends of ten or fifteen years become strangers. Then the years began to slip away one by one, as though they were dead roses being plucked from the vine. My name was an earlier memory retained a little while longer but eventually it, too, was "plucked from the vine." And then we were down to the very, very early memories of her childhood which manage to linger for quite some time.

The process can be quite confusing and frustrating for all parties. But there is another key to the survival on this one. Just go with the flow. I can't tell you how many name changes and name stories we have to tell. But as time went on, all family members and friends just got used to it. I made a special effort to let folks know what was happening and I didn't want anyone getting upset and more importantly, I didn't want anyone upsetting my Mother with their attempts at corrections.

But, I think, the best "name" story is the one regarding my husband. His name is Mark. He came into my life about the second year my Mother was in the throes of this disease. Although she apparently had no problem in the beginning with his name, as the years went by it became harder and harder for her to remember his name. The most important thing to keep in mind during all of this is that old memories will stick. New experiences will not. And the old memories seem to overtake and/or replace any new experiences. It's tough in the beginning, but once you get the motion here, it is easy to distinguish and decipher what is going on in their head.

As the years went on my husband, Mark, became Charlie, who was a high school friend that I dated for about two years while in high school. Which, by the way, was about 35 years earlier. And, of course, the similarities were there. Blond hair, blue eyes, medium build, etc., so you can understand how and why she might make that connection. When my husband would come home, he would say, "Hi, honey! Hi, Mom!" And she would say, "Hi, Charlie!" Well, not only did he and the rest of us get used to it, but quite often, in jest, we would refer to my husband, Mark, as Charlie.

One day he came home and did his usual greeting of "Hi, honey! Hi, Mom!" and my Mother responded, "Hi, Floyd!" We all looked confused as we scampered our eyes around the room and at each other. *Floyd!?!?* We tried desperately to control ourselves so as not to hurt her feelings. No one spoke a word. We just accepted it and went about our business. But that night, when she went to bed and we were sitting in the family room watching TV, during a commercial it was as though a psychic bolt went through the room. All of us looked up and at each other at exactly the same moment and realized the same thought was running through all our minds. We whispered simultaneously, *"Floyd?!"* And our quiet laughter became uncontrollable. We still wonder to this day who her mystery man, Floyd, might be. My husband, Mark, had become Floyd and poor Charlie was lost in the shuffle!

We know it's not particularly nice to laugh at people who have disabilities, but at times the spontaneous levity has managed to lighten the spirits just a bit. And laughing is probably not the best way to describe our feelings or actions. It's just that sometimes she could be so damn cute even in the midst of this devastating experience, you couldn't help but muster up a giggle or two and just melt with love. The important thing to remember here, again, is do not reprimand any mistakes or try to make corrections. It simply confuses the situation and upsets them more than they already are. Go with the flow and let the names abound! Whoever or whatever you're called or anyone else, just go with it! Let everyone else know that this is on the horizon and tell them not to be upset if their names aren't remembered. Who knows? You might like the change.

Chapter 5

"You pray that this is only a joke . . ."

Your Plunge Into The Sea of Darkness

Yes, you pray. You deny. You make excuses to yourself and everyone else. But as the days and weeks slip by and you can no longer run from the truth, your own thoughts become confused and chaotic. If you remember the first time in your life that you ever experienced any kind of trauma or disappointment, you remember how the pit of your stomach seemed bottomless and your throat didn't swallow any more. There is an emotion inside you that is so foreign, you think that you, yourself, have some kind of mental malfunction. A panic creeps in that is so intense it feels like your skin is going to explode.

You pray for sleep at night, and when you wake up, you pray for the day to end, hoping that this "joke" is only going to last one more day and that the next day everything will be fresh and new and okay. In the beginning, know and recognize one thing, and one thing only. This is no joke and it won't be okay in the morning.

I know. I should be writing warm and fuzzy thoughts of support and reinforcement and good things so you can go forthright into this battle with your sword drawn and a big smile on your face. But the best thing I can do for you right now is to let you in on the absolute truth. Because with the truth, you can tackle whatever lies before you with strength, perseverance and knowledge. I tell no tales here and I cover up nothing. So-called experts may not like what I have to say, but when those experts have walked in my shoes, then they can take my hand and we will walk together and perhaps shed a tear or two with each other *for* each other.

The best thing you can do for yourself is to face head on what the future holds. And go forward with the strength that you know you have, because, you see, this is a journey for two. And you are the leader, you are the guide, the teacher, the consoler. You must have the strength and you must show your strength. Do yourself a favor and recognize that strength early on and grab hold of whatever imaginary sword you can find. Because the battle is right before your eyes and you are the warrior. But guess what? With careful planning, careful preparation, your strength, your perseverance and all the knowledge you suck from whatever sources you need to go to, you can survive.

There are little keys and clues all along the way. Little keys and clues that I will try to remember and pass on to you, willingly and lovingly. Our closed little club here is rather hidden and obscure from the rest of the world but trust me, there are hundreds of thousands of us out there. Each one feeling extraordinarily alone and helpless. REACH OUT! It may appear to be a hidden and closed club, but once you make the connection, a whole new world opens up and there you are. Right smack in the middle of all those new friends who are surviving and more than willing to take your hand and help you walk the path.

You no longer have to "take that plunge into the sea of darkness" all by yourself. The plunge will simply be rolling up your sleeves and doing what you know you have to do. It doesn't have to be dark and you don't have to be alone. Be open, be honest, be candid with yourself, your victim, and all those around you. Make them understand and make them aware.

I told you earlier that this was no joke. But in reality, this is one of life's little jokes that continues to prop itself right smack in the middle of our existence. It's another hurdle. It's another test. We've been there before. Perhaps a different circumstance, a different time. But one thing we do know for sure, they keep coming and our job is to get through them. Our job is face it and go onward.

Further on, I will discuss how important it is going to be for all of us to begin our campaign. We MUST be the catalyst for HealthCare reform for our elders in this country. And there is going to be another group that's not going to like the things I have to say in this book. And that group is our legislators and our congressman. But there again, when that group walks in my shoes, and lived my experience with this life altering affliction, then I want to hear what they have to say. They don't seem to be adversely bothered with these types of problems because this is the group that retires with full salaries and benefits and who can afford some of the devastatingly expensive care. They have a way of either sweeping the entire problem under the carpet or ignoring us, hoping we'll go away. Trust me, I'm not going away.

This is part of that "sea of darkness" that I speak of. The more rules and regulations they put on those who have nowhere to go and do not have the financial resources to "float" through, the more ways people figure out how to circumvent the system and the rules. The more they take away from us or disallow, the more ways we figure out how to make it work. It can be over-whelming, but with careful and clever planning, not impossible. Perhaps with enough people who skirt the rules and the more attention we bring to this devastation, we can finally get someone's attention and get the kind of assistance that is so desperately needed. When I get through with this book, there will not be one secret not revealed and many wounds opened. *Someone* will have to take notice.

Chapter 6

" . . . journey through timelessness and spacelessness."

Bedknobs and Broomsticks and Bedsheets

I hate to keep repeating myself, but sometimes it's necessary. Over and over I've said how important it is to not reprimand or attempt to correct any mistakes. Don't question any statements, no matter how outrageous or bizarre they may seem. There are things that go on in the minds of Alzheimer's victims that would send any of us over the edge. So don't think that they are not teetering on the brink every second of every minute of every hour of their terrorized existence. It is our job to attempt to take the terror out of that existence and replace it with as much love and understanding as is humanly possible.

And it's not just hallucinations that create the terror. Or a thought that comes racing through their minds that creates the terror. Their terror can exist in the mere idea of doing something wrong or, as their memory begins to noticeably fade and they recognize that fact, the terror of <u>forgetting</u> to do something is always present. Remember, when folks begin to age, there are years and years of conditioned responses all bundled up inside there somewhere. And when those conditioned responses begin to show themselves, it's always at the wrong time in the wrong place and for the wrong reason. DO NOT REPRIMAND! DO NOT CORRECT! Sometimes this becomes very difficult as *our* conditioned response is to correct when we see that an error has been committed. Let me give you some examples.

When the time came that I had to take complete control for my Mother's welfare and she finally had to move in with me, I quit my job and fully intended to stay home with her and tend to her. She was still quite mobile then but certainly in no condition to be left alone. So, we hung around the house doing house things and garden things, etc.

I usually had a few house cleaning projects that I scheduled each day for myself. This was because we had a huge house and it just simply could not be fully cleaned in one day. So, the best plan was to rotate house duties on a daily basis. One day the kitchen, the next day the family room, etc. Well, this particular day was the bedroom day. I had cleaned all four bedrooms upstairs and changed the sheets on all beds. And my sweet Mother was right there along side of me, helping me every inch of the way. I had stacked the dirty sheets by the staircase and when we were done, I grabbed all the dirty sheets and ran them down stairs to the laundry room. While I was down there, I got a phone call that lasted maybe two or three minutes. When I went back upstairs, she had stripped all the beds of the clean sheets and had them stacked by the staircase!

My first instinct was to get hysterical and start screaming about all the work that had just been undone. My first words were "Oh my god, what did you do?!" I saw a look of sheer terror and disbelief come over her and I wanted to slap myself, once again, for jumping into a response before thinking. My next thought was "Oh my god, shut up, you stupid fool! Can't you see what you've done to her?!" I quickly calmed down and took her by the hand and simply picked up the sheets and we proceeded to redo the beds. I told her that what had happened was my fault and she was only doing the right thing. I hugged her and thanked her for being such a good housekeeper.

But do you understand the thought process here? We had done the beds. The dirty sheets had been taken downstairs. She remembered something about clean sheets and dirty sheets and changing the sheets, but couldn't quite put the whole package together. So her old-time, years long, conditioned response took hold, and her remaining thought was to do her usual housewife duty and change the sheets on the bed by first stripping off the existing sheets!

Another problem we encountered along the way solved itself in a very unusual manner. At dinnertime, as I prepared the food and scurried about the kitchen, I would grab a minute or two to set the table. Then I'd go back to working with the food and the next thing I knew, my Mother was clearing all the dishes off the table a putting them back in the cabinets. Again, a bad response from me. I know it probably sounds like I'm a hysterical maniac and react adversely every time my Mother did something. Well, I'm not hysterical nor am I a maniac, but admittedly, in the beginning, my reactions were not great. But, with patience and the growing knowledge of these experiences, I began to calm down and take everything in stride and find alternative solutions to these problems.

Anyway, this table setting fiasco went on for a while and finally I discovered a solution. I gave my Mother the initial job of setting the table. Several times a night! I would ask her to set the table. Somewhere in the next ten minutes she would "unset" the table. I'd wait about five more minutes, and then ask her to set the table. Ten minutes later she'd "unset" the table. You get the picture. I was getting the table set and if it was suddenly "unset", it was not my work and effort that was being undone. And she was reacting to her conditioned responses. Setting, clearing. Setting, clearing. Everybody was happy.

So these are just a few examples. But my point here is that you have to learn a new attitude and a new response mechanism. Spouses seem to have the most difficulty with the changes and the adjustment. They are the ones who have spent a lifetime with the victim on a daily basis and who are currently experiencing a 24-hour disruption in routine, memory failure, and the many problems that begin to occur with this disease. Watching their loved one begin to fail and to see confusion overtake logic is frightening and sad and acceptance is most difficult.

The important key here is to go with the flow. Each person is different and each experience will be different according to the life patterns that the victim has set and lifestyles that the victim is accustomed to. Their "journey through timelessness and spacelessness" can be terror filled and confusing or you can ease the anxiety for them by simply making these "mistakes" a part of their routine and ignoring the fact that there was an error made at all. Your job is to cool your jets and put your imagination to work seeking alternative solutions using the "bedknobs and broomsticks" approach by simply figuring out another way to do it!

The emphasis here, again, is DO NOT CORRECT! DO NOT REPRIMAND! Keep their anxiety level to a minimum with your love and acceptance of everything they do.

Chapter 7

". . . squeezing until you can no longer fight."

Spirit

This is a good spot to interject one of the biggest factors in anyone's survival of anything that comes your way. I've learned this lesson many times over in my own personal life and have tried to convey the message and the experiences to friends and family so they may benefit from it. Some get it. Some don't. There are a few people out there in the entertainment industry that do extraordinarily well in their efforts to give something to the American public in terms of hope and support through their venues of television talk shows. Leeza Gibbons does a smashing job on her true-to-life segments of family trauma and comeback and her message to never give up hope. Montel Williams, also, does a terrific job on his show with real situations and his constant giving of help to those who seem lost. But there is something going on currently in the media which is so heartwarming and exciting that I wish I could be a part of it every single day. There is someone out there conveying a message to millions of people without screaming repentance and damnation because you've made a few mistakes.

The individual that I call a darling of the media, and currently taking first spot in my heart, Oprah Winfrey, has a segment on her show called "Remembering Your Spirit." I recall a few years ago when Oprah made the very wise decision to change the format of her show because she was not happy with where it was going based on the direction of the talk show genre, in general. She has, since, created a venue of such high quality and needed information that she leaves all others in the dust.

But the "spirit" segment has always and continues to be the grandest of inspirational support for folks of all walks of life and all types of situations where they need help and guidance. Let us use this same type of inspirational support here in our current situation.

Remember what I said in Chapter 5 when I spoke of your job as teacher and consoler, the leader and guide through this journey of darkness. And, yes, I know. You're first reaction is to shrink back and say, "That's not me she's talking about!" Well, guess what? It certainly is you that I'm talking about.

You have within you, albeit, hidden somewhere, the spirit of survival. A spirit so strong that sometimes it can click in without you even knowing it and there you are. Weeks, months, years down the line living in the middle of what may seem to have been a hopeless situation, surviving like a gladiator in the midst of the biggest battle of his life. But, you say, I don't feel that spirit.

Well, know one thing. Your spirit comes from your power. And your power is God given. It is his gift to you. It is his same power. It is HIS power. When you shirk, when you shrink, when you agonize, you lose your power. Consistently and absolutely. But the more you push forward, the more you meet it head on, the stronger your power becomes and the grander your spirit grows!

Remember to have faith in all things, especially yourself. You don't have to drop to your knees in prayer every day and you don't have to tithe your money away. You don't have to hang religious artifacts all over your house and you don't have to run to a temple of worship every week. If you believe in your own power and accept that you have that power and act on it, that is all that God asks of you. Because that power will get you through all things and guide you to make the right decisions and guide you in your interactions with all people. Acknowledge his gift by using your power, his power.

As you struggle through in the beginning of your current situation, you will go forward as the blind man taking his first step with his new cane. You will feel the boa constrictor of hopelessness squeezing and squeezing until you *think* you can no longer fight. But as you keep plodding along, and giving out your love and compassion, you will discover that your power begins to manifest itself in your spirit. Suddenly, like a lotus flower opening for the first time, light will come, answers will come, help will come.

That's not to say that you can just sit on your happy little butt and expect everything to come your way. My message here is to move forward and accept what is before you. Meet it with determination and strength. Keep your spirit flowing by recognizing that it has appeared. It belongs to you and is simply waiting for your direction. The more you give, the more you get. Your spirit wants to grow. It wants to double and triple itself on your behalf. Don't let it down.

Chapter 8

"... fear of discovery."

More Subtle Signals

DEPRESSION

There are, of course, going to be many, many signs in the beginning that are going to give you clues that trouble is on the horizon. But one of the more important signs that you need to be aware of are hints of depression. This is one of the frightening aspects of this disease and leads many people to suicide. I don't mean to frighten you un-necessarily, but the last thing that any person needs to cope with is a suicide. Having experienced it among friends, I can't imagine having a family member succumb to such depths and then, having to live with a guilt that I may have noticed something, but didn't.

Depression can rear it's ugly head in so many different ways, it may be hard to detect, but one thing is for sure. You need to look deeply into the behavior of the victim and try to distinguish whether or not you're dealing with actual depression or simply mood swings, or just the strange aspects and behavior of the disease. If you think you can't make any determination, by all means, seek help from your physician or a therapist.

My Mother really didn't experience much depression, but later on, my Father, as he began to grow older and began, also, to show signs of the disease, grew increasingly more depressed as the weeks went by. My parents had always traveled back and forth from Illinois to Florida, spending winters in the South and summers up North. When my Father was no longer able to care for my Mother, she came to live with me full time while my Father stayed in Florida for the winters. His last winter there, he quietly sunk into a depression that went completely unnoticed and undetected by all those around him. I certainly wasn't aware that anything was wrong merely because of the distance between us even though I spoke to him three to four times a week.

I finally received a call from some of his neighbors who took it upon themselves to look in on him and then call me with a report. He had gone into such a deep depression that he became a recluse. He hadn't bathed in weeks or changed his clothes, hadn't cleaned the house, gone food shopping or eaten meals. His hair was grown down to his shoulders, his beard completely grown out and he had lost approximately 60 pounds. I was shocked at the report and deeply saddened when I saw him when we picked him up at the airport. We took him home and started cleaning him up and most importantly, getting him back to a healthy condition. We were able to put the 60 pounds back on him and bring him around and back into shape.

I spoke with our physician about the situation and asked him how this could happen and how anyone could get into this condition. He simply said that many, many older people go into a depression like that when they're left alone or on their own.

But this brings us back into the discussion of Alzheimer's and depression. Many times the Alzheimer's victim will not go into a depression, but when they do, it is, again, their fear of discovery. They will shut themselves away from the rest of the world hoping that no one will notice and they will not be discovered. The signs can be subtle, but some are not so subtle.

HYGIENE

Keep in mind, that the disease itself is going to bring about a change in habits and behavior. But I've learned from experience that there are certain and very clear signs that designate a depressed state of mind. Hygiene is probably the most prevalent. From the onset, keep an eye on the individuals hygiene habits, i.e., bathing, brushing their teeth, keeping their hair clean, shaving, changing clothes and underwear regularly. If you see extreme changes in these behaviors, it's a good bet that they're sinking and their focus has switched from hygiene to the many areas of confusion that this disease will take them and straight into the ever-dreaded "fear of discovery." That is why it is so important to be above board and candid with the individual. They may continue to deny that anything is wrong, but with loving reinforcement every single day, their fear can subside and chances are the depression will leave or, if you're lucky, never grab hold.

Remember, when you or I get depressed, the main reasons for sinking deeper and deeper is because we have no one at the moment to share our anguish because we choose not to share it for fear of bothering or depressing other people. But once we are able to get it out of our system, it seems to lighten the load even for just a tiny bit. It's the same principle here. Knowing that they are not alone and that all is understood with regard to their affliction, it can get better. The important thing is to open the doors of communication.

HIDING VALUABLES

Another sign to look for is hiding money or valuables. Again, a fear takes over that they're going to lose these things or that their valuables are going to be taken away. As a result, they begin to "stash" them all over the place with the intent of getting back to them later. But, of course, because the memory is failing, they forget not only where the hiding places are, but that anything has been hidden at all. When this begins to happen, the best thing to do is to take the valuables and put them in a safe place. This way, everyone knows where they are and nothing will get lost. I can't tell you how many people have told me about lost diamond rings or watches and some, to this day, have not found them. I have a friend that is still looking for her Mother's wedding rings as she would like to have had them for a remembrance, but has no idea where they are because her Mother "hid" them some time ago.

When my Father began to clear out the house in Florida because he knew we were going to be selling it, he found almost $1000 in small bills stashed in every nook and cranny in the house. There was money stuffed in books, magazines, under drawer liners, Kleenex boxes, you name it. We had discovered some time prior to that time that it was necessary to begin taking valuables and money matters out of my Mother's hands, but had no idea of the magnitude of the problem even before we made our discovery and decisions.

It may be difficult to deal with this aspect, because most people don't want to give up their independence and having their own money is independence. But it must be done. Particularly if the individual is still in the beginning stages and can still handle somewhat living on their own. At some point in time, someone is going to have to take over their financial matters. They cannot seem to grasp it any more and bills go unpaid leaving them, at times, in desperate situations. Heaven forbid, a gas bill goes unpaid in the dead of winter and the heat goes off. Not to mention other utilities, insurance and even mortgage payments or taxes. The Alzheimer's Association has recently begun to address this problem for victims who are either still living alone or even in nursing homes. Some of these poor folks do not have family members they can trust or perhaps not available on a regular basis to tend to their financial matters. The Alzheimer's Association has sent out questionnaires asking for people to volunteer their time to these individuals and assist them in their financial dealings and the handling of their money.

The point here is that eventually these functions will have to be taken away and handled by other persons including the day-to-day handling of all cash monies. It may be necessary to allot an amount as small as $5.00 or $10.00 for pin money or emergency telephone money, possibly a little more in case they need to have lunch while their lost! And sometimes, they can be lost for very long times. Scary? Yes. Real? Yes. Impossible? Not at all.

DRIVING

This is another one of those situations where it may become difficult. Driving represents an even bigger stand for independence. Once a person's driving privilege's are taken away, they are completely and totally at the mercy of other individuals for most if not all of their necessities and/or social interaction. They now are dependent on other people for everything from grocery shopping, trips to the post office or hardware store, doctor's visits or pharmacy needs, transportation to and from any social event, or even something as simple as a Sunday drive. The inability to fend for themselves represents aging and incompetence and these two things are probably the hardest for any of us to accept.

But the major problems here are basically the safety of others as well as themselves and the probability that one day they will take off in the car and start driving only to unintentionally end up hundreds of miles from home.

There are several stories I can relate on this subject. For instance, one day while my Father was here in Illinois, he decided he wanted to go to Sears. Unfortunately, there is no Sears in our small town. He was thinking of the Sears in Florida and would have driven God knows where to find it.

My Mother would go grocery shopping and come out to discover that she had forgotten where she parked the car. One day, it took her four hours to find it while my Father sat home waiting and wondering what had happened to her. But I think the best instance is the story of my friend's father who was going to drive to their summer home which was about 350 miles North into Wisconsin. He was found about 200 miles west somewhere close to the Iowa state line. So this gives you an idea of the types of situations that can happen and the problems that may be encountered where directions and destinations are concerned.

But the safety factor is probably the biggest issue when we discuss driving. The actual mechanics are the danger we speak of and are not difficult to understand. When the memory begins to fade, so do the motor functions, thinking processes and the ability to use logic. The brake pedal becomes the acceleration pedal and vice versa. The functions on the drive shaft, i.e. drive, reverse, park, etc. no longer make sense. And the ability to distinguish what a red light or green light means has dissipated. These things alone are major factors in the safety issue.

But there are still other factors that can contribute to the danger. Speed no longer is of any consequence. They will decide to do 25 in a 65 mph zone. Signaling for turns or turning from the correct lane no longer becomes a necessary function. And stopping at intersections is a huge, huge problem. Even though they see the stop sign, they simply forget what it means and forget to stop.

As I stated, this is probably the number one problem when it comes to taking away privileges or responsibilities. I've seen television documentaries where a camera was attached to the back seat of an elderly victim's auto and he was taped while taking a five minute drive. In those five minutes, he could have been responsible for no less than SIX major accidents on the road. But when he saw the tape of himself driving and was asked if he was willing to give up his keys, he stated emphatically NO, he was not.

Sometimes this becomes not an issue for discussion or negotiation but simply something that MUST be done for the safety of all concerned. It may turn ugly and you may have to deal with it for several weeks, but it is your duty as a responsible citizen or spouse, or son or daughter to take the initiative and see to it that this danger does not present itself by someone from your family. If a very serious accident is caused by the individual who should not have been driving, and other persons are seriously injured or worse, killed, the financial repercussions can be devastating to your family. And the emotional repercussions of being responsible for the death of an individual in someone else's family, is life long. Especially if you could have prevented it by being responsibly insistent and simply taken away the car keys.

Chapter 9

". . . corruption of mind, body and soul."

As Time Goes By

As we get passed the early stages and fate drives us further into the trenches, there will come many new problems and situations that need to be confronted and dealt with on a regular basis. People often comment that caring for an Alzheimer's victim is like caring for a two-year old. This is far from the truth. A two-year old can be taught and will eventually learn whatever it is that we must teach our infants to become full functioning human beings. Our poor victims will not only never be able to learn anything new, they will forget most of their human bodily and mental functions and become helpless and almost fetal like in their existence. As each day passes, one more thing will become impossible for them to do and their adult thought process dwindles down to almost nothing and then finally, nothing.

ACCIDENTS

We, as caregivers, must see to their most basic needs and keep a watchful eye to see that they don't, in some bizarre way, harm themselves or others with the most innocent of objects. A drinking glass can become a lethal weapon. A one-step ladder can become their killer. You've heard of people who "child-proof" their houses for their own children or for visiting children. You will have to "Alzheimer's proof" your house to keep your loved one safe. I will list here as many areas as I can remember that can cause possible harm or damage in your home.

1. The bath or shower - this is an area that may require some special installations or the purchase of some rather inexpensive equipment. As the ability to move limbs grows more difficult, you will need some handles and bars attached to the walls of your bath. It becomes very difficult to make these steps into the tub for a bath or shower without some assistance. And don't forget the non-skid rubber mat in the bathtub. Also, there are small, inexpensive "shower chairs" available that will enable the individual to actually sit in the tub without having to get all the way down into it. Once down, getting back up sometimes becomes a torturous ordeal. If you have a shower stall in your bathroom, this is a little easier, but remember to put a non-skid rubber mat on the floor of your

shower with a hole cut out around the drain. Skids and fall-downs can happen there, also.

2. Staircases - ascending or descending staircases can be treacherous. Always have handrails on your staircases and if, possible, keep some kind of gate at the top and bottom so access is virtually impossible. This may not become a problem early on, but later when walking and even standing is becoming difficult, they will still try and use the stairs to go out of the house.

3. Carpentry or garden tools - needless to say, electric carpentry tools are out of the question. Many male victims who have had woodworking shops in their basements or who have been wonderful handymen around the house, think they can still perform these duties. Perhaps in the beginning, but "as time goes by", these tools will become exceedingly dangerous in their hands. Any number of things can go wrong, including forgetting to keep fingers and hands out of the way of drills, saws, hammers, etc. Be smart and be safe. Get rid of them. Gardening tools are another danger along with knitting and crochet tools. Eventually the skill will be gone altogether and the necessity for having these tools will be gone also. Keep a watchful eye on a daily basis so you can determine when these tools need to be extracted from the area.

4. Cooking - this has been probably one of the most dangerous areas in the Alzheimer's community. I cannot tell you how many times my Mother would attempt to start dinner and left everything on the stove burning to a crisp and, at times, having fires erupt as a result. If the individual is still living at home (which they really shouldn't be at this stage), a good idea would be to have the stove disconnected and get a microwave if there isn't already one in the house. Actually, by this time, the individual should be living with another relative so this issue doesn't come up. Stoves and cooking and the fires that develop from them are the ultimate destruction. When you are in the throes of dealing with an Alzheimer's victim, you don't need to deal with home reconstruction or possible injuries or death that can result from this kind of accident.

5. Lighting - as the caregiver, it will ultimately be your responsibility to see that there is sufficient lighting installed in all major areas of the house, i.e., staircases, bathroom and bathroom shower stalls, closets, sharp or crowded corners, etc. to alleviate the danger of falls or bruising caused by miscalculated steps or turns.

6. Smoking - this, also, can be particularly dangerous. If the victim is a smoker, close, and I

mean *close*, attention must be given to their habits. I have found partially smoked cigarettes that had been butted out by hand in my Mother's lingerie drawers. This was **after** we had taken all cigarettes, lighters and matches away from her and diligently began monitoring her smoking habits. Unfortunately, we had other smokers in the house and she would sneak cigarettes out of their packs, hide them in her room and later in the evening, have a puff or two and then put it out and hide it in her lingerie drawer! Another potential danger for home fires and exhaustive destruction. But the other danger on this level is lit cigarettes left in ashtrays because they forgot they were there and walked away from it. That's the reason for paying close attention and then, ultimately, the necessity for monitoring all smoking. Eventually, the best of all worlds would be to have them quit altogether. We know this is difficult, but eventually, the habit itself will be forgotten.

DAILY FUNCTIONS

As I have stated previously, daily functions that we take for granted every single day, become almost insurmountable tasks or leave the memory banks altogether. It becomes the caregiver's responsibility to see that these functions are handled and kept a part of the daily routine. The victim, relatively early on, will look at some of these functions as completely foreign actions. They won't remember how to dress themselves, eat with a fork, how to bathe themselves, or even change underwear on a regular basis. Everything becomes a problem and you are the one that has to take responsibility for them.

1. Dressing will probably be the first noticeable problem. You will begin to see a change in dress style or a lack of completion in certain dressing tasks such as tied shoelaces, sweaters or blouses or shirts not completely buttoned, etc. The change in dress style can be a shock, at times. For instance, if someone was a fastidious dresser and was able to mix and match with any degree of fashion or style, you may find that this ability has gone by the wayside. You may begin to see pink sweaters with red skirts or plaids and stripes. Again, the gentle approach is the best approach. I would see my Mother come down the stairs with some really questionable outfits, but I would gently take her by the hand and "suggest" that maybe we could find something that would be more appropriate for "the weather." In the process, I was able to redress her with some degree of style and completion of tasks. Because we had always had candid discussions about her disease, my Mother was aware that dressing herself had become a problem. Being the jokester

and wonderfully humorous person that she was, one day she came down with my Father's size 13 gym shoes, a knee-length nightgown, and a winter hat with furry ear muffs that she left dangling around her ears and simply said "I'm ready!" and presented herself to all that could see. We all laughed and laughed and even took a picture. She got the biggest kick of all because she made us all laugh! But remember that as time goes by, both the mental and physical concept of dressing is going to be a confusing process to the victim and you, once again, must be there to assist.

2. Hygiene is, yet again, mentioned and will also be a very noticeable and continuing problem. With women it can be a little easier as women seem to have a greater sensibility about their own hygiene. Men, on the other hand, being the "hunter warriors" don't seem to experience the same concern or sensibility. But in either case, you will need to watch this closely. I've heard of cases where someone will discover that the victim hasn't bathed in five or six weeks and, as you know, this can become extremely noticeable because along with the lack of bathing or showering, is the lack of clean underwear. The same with shampooing one's hair or even shaving. Again, a sensitive issue but one that must be confronted and dealt with. With my Mother, it was simply taking her by the hand and putting her

in the bathtub. With my Father, it was much more difficult but yet manageable. It finally became an issue of pride in his case. He was always known for being a snappy dresser and looking his best, so I just let his own pride get the best of him and he would finally succumb and get himself into the shower.

3. Another very, very sensitive issue is incontinence. Remember in my outline I made mention of the fact that you need to consider this problem very early on because it comes on faster than you think. This, again, can be a difficult one to tackle. But there are many reasons why you need to pay special attention here because one day everything appears to be okay, and then the next day you have an embarrassing situation confronting you head on with no warning and no preparation. It is, of course, embarrassing for you, but it can be excruciatingly embarrassing for the victim. I have experienced wet clothing, soaked car seats (mine and others), soaked furniture (mine and others), or the appearance of this devilish experience in public places. Truly, most folks are quite understanding especially in this day and age of the publicity given this disease and all dementia of older persons. But it is still embarrassing to the victim and can affect them in some pretty terrible ways. They will refuse to leave the house. This includes not only shopping or appointments, but

all social functions or family gatherings. You need to confront the problem, discuss it, and get them into full fitted plastic briefs to replace their regular underpants as quickly as possible. Also, I got into the habit of taking a bag along containing extra briefs, plastic bags, wipettes, washcloth and soap, a towel, and a change of clothing. Just as you would take a bag along for an infant or a child, we are now in the time of this disease which requires the same attendance. Don't be afraid to deal with this. Confronting it and being prepared is much easier than being caught off guard and being embarrassed or having to cut short a visit because hygiene has become a priority.

4. Eating - one would think that eating should not be a problem because when one gets hungry, one will simply eat. This is not the case. I'm not exactly sure what happens, but either they don't get hungry, or my best guess is that perhaps the feeling of hunger has now become a foreign feeling and they can't remember what to do to alleviate it. At any rate, the daily function of eating now becomes your daily function of feeding. If they are still on their own, chances are they will not be eating properly. I know many people who have had to set up the Meals on Wheels program or make it their business to take meals that they cooked at home over to the

victim's house. If the victim is living with you, the regular mealtime, more than likely, will not be a problem. However, "as time goes by", there will still be many problems connected to the eating and feeding process. At first, my Mother was okay with eating at the table with the rest of us. Then she got to the point where she would just play with her food and we had to prod her along the entire meal to get her to eat. Then we encountered the cutting of the meat where she could no longer remember how to cut and we had to do it for her. Then some rather difficult problems developed. She could chew her food, but could no longer remember to swallow. That function, or process, was leaving her memory, so she would "squirrel" her food or tuck it into her cheeks and it would never get swallowed. We finally had to change her diet to stews and chopped meats until finally, we are at the pureed or baby food stage. Even this is becoming difficult as the function of swallowing is becoming more and more foreign to her. Eventually, the whole process of eating is going to completely leave the memory and you will have to begin spoonfeeding. Again, this is an area that you will absolutely be facing and although it isn't a pleasant thought, it's better to have the knowledge and at least be somewhat prepared for what the future holds. It is also a good idea to make sure that you include in the diet some kind of food supplement, such as Ensure. These are milkshake-like liquids that are especially manufactured to hold the maximum of vitamins and minerals to supplement the diet and insure that the individual is getting the proper nutritional benefits. I make sure that my Mother's meals consist of all the necessary food groups, even in baby food form, and I make sure that she gets some kind of strained or pureed fruit snack each morning and afternoon. You also need to keep an eye out for dehydration. Since they will probably not remember to take care of it themselves, you will need to see to it that they get at least three to four good glasses of water each day.

5. Exercise - here again is a daily function that will be left by the wayside. As we have all been preached to all our lives, exercise is vital to our health. Unfortunately, there are very few of us who actually pay attention to this advice. However, even at this juncture with this disease, exercise can be extremely healthful. It can aid in oxygen for the body and help ward off bone deterioration or certain forms of arthritis, aid in keeping the heart healthy, etc. If you only walk for a half hour a day, it can be most helpful. If you can take the time to do a few aerobic exercises in the house, this is even better. Fifteen minutes a day of arm swinging, knee lifts, walking in place, or whatever you can dream up can do

wonders not only for the health, but for the mental attitude as well. Make sure that the same time each day is set aside and the same amount of time is spent. Also, if you can put together a little routine, that would be wonderful, but remember to keep the routine the same day after day. In other words, if you swing arms first, remember to do that first each and every day. And so on. The routine and structure is going to be beneficial in that there will be no changes to upset or confuse. If they become confined to a wheelchair, even lifting arms can be helpful. Remember, it keeps the oxygen flowing.

These are just a few of the areas that I wanted to bring to your attention. There will be countless more, I am sure, but these seem to be some of the more prevalent and immediate ones. Remember what I said earlier about taking care of a child. It is much more stressful than that. As the days and weeks go by, there will be more and more that will be lost to the victim and, subsequently, more and more that you will have to take responsibility for. Again, gentleness is the key here and although it is going to become more and more difficult for you and more and more stressful, love and compassion will ease the pain and anxiety for your loved one and "as time goes by", it will open the gates of understanding for you.

Chapter 10

" . . . when the invasion begins.. "

Flying Polar Bears

Along with the planning, signs and signals, and daily functions, there is another area that most people are totally unprepared for. We begin, now, to discuss the total dementia of this disease and your part in handling the strange and bizarre. I also mentioned that there may be times when humor and levity will play a part in this transition. You will learn that, at times, it may be difficult to hold yourself back from a good guffaw now and then. This is perfectly alright. Laughter is always better received than any other emotion or statement in this instance and even though they may not be understanding what your laughing about, they may laugh right along with you simply because it feels good. Laughter denotes happiness and if people are happy, then everything must be alright. I began, early on, to document certain situations that I encountered and realized as I would read through my notes, how funny and cute some of them were. Of course, there were some pretty bizarre ones also, but the important thing to remember, again and always, is love and compassion and understanding.

HALLUCINATIONS

My dear sweet Mother had a way about her that, even though she was in the middle of this horrific disease, was able to bring about a smile, a giggle, a fall-down hysterical fit of laughter to all of us. I already mentioned her imp-like humor in her dressing up in funny outfits, but even beyond that she was able to keep us smiling.

About eight years ago, my husband and I built a rather large house in Illinois. Even though it was only he and I, our intention was to build a home large enough to eventually house us AND my Mother and my Father. The purpose for this was because we knew that my Mother had been stricken with Alzheimer's and eventually she would be with us full-time and then, soon thereafter, my Father would have to come. This house certainly was not imbedded in my Mother's memory since it was a new home. But they would come to live with us during the summers and would be their home away from home.

We were all still able to go out for dinner and shopping together, but one particular night, all four of us decided to go out for dinner. Upon our return, we began to pull in the driveway to the house and my Mother said, "Who lives here?" And I said, "We do, Mom." And her response was, "*You do?!* Oh, honey, I'm so proud of you!" And we hugged.

A few nights later we went out for dinner again. Upon our return, we pulled in the driveway and my Mother said, "Who lives here?" And I said, "We do, Mom." And her response was "*You do?!* Oh, honey, I'm so proud of you?" And so on and so on. This continued until she was no longer able to leave the house.

There are other areas in the mind tricks category that are not so pleasant or cute, but nevertheless, they have to be dealt with. I think one of the most horrific for my Mother was the "dead bodies" encounter. One night while I was preparing dinner, I noticed that my Mother was sort of skulking around the house and peeking around corners before she would enter a room. We had kind of a circular set up between the kitchen, family room, living room, and dining room. So she could walk the circle and end up right back by me. But this particular night, as I said, she was acting stranger than usual. I approached her and put my hands on her shoulders and asked her what was wrong. She, of course, told me nothing was wrong, but I knew better. Then I said, "Mom, I know something is wrong. I'm here to help you and you can tell me anything. I won't laugh and I won't be mad. Why don't you tell me and see if I can help?" Well, she did. She told me that she was afraid to enter certain rooms because of the bodies that were lying on the floors! I asked her if they were alive or dead. She said they were half and half! I wasn't sure if she meant that half of them were alive and half of them were dead, or if they were all half-dead and half-alive. But I figured it best not to dwell on the negative aspect of this particular hallucination.

I wrestled with a solution for about ten seconds and finally said, "Oh, those bodies! I see them sometimes, too." And she said "YOU DO?" And I proceeded, "Yes, I do. But do you know what I do. I just kick them aside and continue walking. Because you see they can't get up, so if I just kick them, they disappear." So she looked down, gave a few kicks and then looked up at me. She said, "You're right, they go away!" So she spent the night kicking away, but we never encountered that particular problem again.

And there is another interesting story that was related to me by a home care nurse. There was a woman that she cared for who, one day, began flinging her arms above her head and continued doing this throughout the day. The nurse finally asked her what the problem was. Was she being bothered by bugs? The woman said, "No! It's those damn flying polar bears. They won't stay out of my hair!" The nurse, also wrestling with a solution for about ten seconds, went into the kitchen and got a can of room spray. She taped a label on the can that read "Flying Polar Bear Repellent" and gave it to the woman who proceeded to spray the room. She kept the spray along side of her continually and was able to successfully ward off her flying polar bears. They never flew through her hair again!

So you get the story. There are going to be any number of hallucinations that are going to come your way. Some funny, some not so funny. But here, again, is where you need to use the "bedknobs and broomsticks" approach. In other words, use your imagination. And, again, do not reprimand or correct. Learn to go with the flow and help out whenever you can. The hallucinations won't go away, but the fear and anxiety of "being discovered" might. And if it takes just kicking a dead body or two or supplying some Flying Polar Bear Repellent to help, so be it.

SEXUAL BEHAVIOR

This subject is always tough for people to face head on or, especially, to discuss. An individual with any form of dementia is not always going to change their sexual behavior or go into some bizarre sexual state of mind. You may not ever have any kind of a sexual behavior incident in your particular situation, but if you do, handle it like you would handle any of the other situations, with patience and understanding.

I remember one night when I had some guests for dinner. My Mother had been fed much earlier and went to bed her regular time. About 10:00 p.m., she marched downstairs in her bra and panties and presented herself in the living room. Admittedly, it was kind of shocking, but all my guests were most understanding, no one said a word, and I just took her by the hand and walked her back to bed.

I heard of a story where an elderly gentleman, in the middle of the night, crawled into his 15-year-old granddaughter's bed. This was not an issue of sexual abuse as these kinds of things did not go on in this family. The granddaughter was well aware of her grandfather's condition and state of mind. And, the interesting part is that the granddaughter was the spitting image of her grandmother, her grandfather's wife. The grandfather was, in his mind, simply getting into bed with his wife. The granddaughter simply got up and took Grandpa by the hand and took him back to his own bed, where he stayed for the rest of the night and never went back to her room or her bed. Her parents were somewhat upset, fearing that she would be upset. Her comments to her parents were quite enlightening to them. She said, "Grandpa used to tuck me in bed. I guess now it's my turn."

I've also heard of people fondling themselves in public or attempting to disrobe, or any number of things that people can do that might be related as sexual.

These kinds of incidents could be construed as bizarre sexual behavior. But remember that these folks are not aware mostly of what they are doing and most behavior does not come from a conscious state of mind. There intent is not necessarily a sexual one, but merely another phase of confusion. Reprimanding is not going to help. You need to clear your head of all preconceived ideas of what sexual behavior should or should not be. Don't be shocked or dismayed at what you may see or experience. This behavior comes from another place amidst mental confusion and is not, in any way, a disorder or intended for any purpose other than a reaching out for a connection to something remembered. A human being's complete expression of love is a sexual encounter and somehow connects us to a full understanding of our emotions. That is their only intent. To somehow understand what is going on in their confused state and oncoming loss of self. A gentle discussion of unacceptable behavior is in order here. Even if you have to do it repeatedly. A reprimand is only going to make matters worse and may even perpetuate or increase the behavior. Your goal is to diminish and eventually eradicate the behavior altogether and to do it as delicately as possible.

Chapter 11

" . . . that glimmer in her eye . . . "

The Happy Wanderer

There is one particular phase of this disease that is going to create sheer terror for you if you don't begin to handle it from the very beginning. As the mind begins to deteriorate and the victim becomes more and more confused, an anxiety sets in. I believe there are several factors that contribute or cause this anxiety. You must remember that the individual has probably led an active life either personally or professionally and will cling to all activities related to that life. Another theory is that when the confusion begins to set in, there is a desire to move around or travel or keep oneself busy either physically or mentally which they believe may help alleviate the mental confusion. The Alzheimer's Association states, "They become dis-oriented and confused, even in their everyday surroundings and to relieve their panic and regain control of their situation, they go in search of something familiar or reassuring." Either way, there is this issue of anxiety.

There are many, many stories of elder persons with the disease who leave the home and don't return for several days, weeks or months, or until they are found. Somewhere in their troubled mind a thought pops up that they have to go to the hardware store, go to work, pick up children, etc. Whatever the thought, it's enough to motivate them to want to get out of the house and continue on their journey or their mission to do whatever it was that entered their mind. But once they leave the house, they have forgotten what they went out for and begin to roam aimlessly around the area or the city or the countryside.

I told you the story about my friend's father who decided he was going to go to their summer home up in Wisconsin and was found about 200 miles west of Chicago. But this book is about my Mother and I have, yet again, another story to relate to you.

My Father and I planned to have my Mother come up from Florida about December 1st one year to enable my Father to have a little respite from the care of my Mother. I was working full-time and commuting from a Northern suburb into Chicago, so it would be necessary for me to have someone come in from Monday through Friday to stay with my Mother until I arrived home from work. I found a lovely lady named Florence, also retired, who was looking for a little extra work for a little extra money.

On Florence's last Thursday with us, we both had a difficult time with my Mother all day and all night. It seemed that my Mother had somehow gotten in her head that she needed to go into town to pick up "the kids." That would be me and my cousin Patrick. Mind you, we are going back about 46 or 47 years when my cousin Patrick and I were buddies.

Florence had done a fine job for two full weeks. By the way, my Mother could not remember her name, but Florence looked like an old friend of my Mother's named Helen. So Florence became Helen. Finally, on Friday, the last day before my Father was to arrive from Florida, I received a call at work from Florence telling me that when she arrived at the house, she could not find my Mother. I said, "What do you mean, you can't find her?!" Florence said, "I've looked everywhere. She's not here!" I told Florence to look upstairs, downstairs, in the basement, in the garage, in closets, in kitchen cabinets! No Mother!

I then told her to call the County Sheriff's office. I called the Sales Office in our home development area. We called the bus lines. I told Florence to hang tight, I was on my way home. When I arrived home, Florence had a tale to tell me. She went next door to a house that was not completely built, but had workmen working all around it. She said she spoke to one young man who said yes, absolutely he had seen my Mother. In fact, he had given her a ride to the shopping mall because she told him she needed to get a bus into town to pick up "the kids!"

This thought hung in her mind from the day and night before and being the responsible and caring Mother that she always was, she became obsessed about getting into town to pick up those kids! Another phone call was made to the Mall security. Now my own personal panic began to set in. I have lost my Mother! My Mother! I do not know where to find my Mother! Not to mention the fact that the next morning my Father was flying in and I had to pick him up at the airport. "Hi, Dad! Welcome back to Chicago. How was your flight? Oh, by the way, we've lost Mother."

You cannot begin to know how your brain scrambles when you are confronted with this kind of crisis. I had four Sheriff's squads in front of my house, neighbors coming out their doors, children riding up to the house on their bicycles, in general, gathering a rather large crowd.

Finally, Florence said that she was going to go over to the Mall to walk around and see if she could locate her. Our hopes were that she did not, in fact, get onto a bus. The Sheriff's police made a call to the local town police to be on the lookout for her. We were doing our best to cover all our bases to try and cut her off at the pass before she got too far away from us. Florence left and I stayed behind at the house to deal with the police and phone calls that were coming in.

About twenty minutes later, the phone rang. It was Florence. "I've got her!" she screamed into the phone. "We're on our way home!" I collapsed into my seat with tears running down my cheeks. I finally swallowed. Something I hadn't done for about two hours.

Florence and my Mother drove into the driveway. I saw them coming onto the street through my front window and I ran out to the front of the house. There was, by now, a huge crowd and two more squad cars making a total of six. I ran to the car, opened the door as my Mother stepped out from the passenger's side. "Oh, Mom!" I screamed. I grabbed her and hugged her. "I am so glad to see you!" She just looked around at all the commotion and then looked at me questioningly and said, "What's going on here?" By now, I was close to hysterics.

"Oh, Mom! All these police are here for you! All these people are here for you! We lost you and couldn't find you. Everyone was looking for you and very, very worried!" She just looked around again in both directions, waved her hand at me and said "Oh, go on." She turned and padded her tiny little feet up the walk to the door, turned again and said, "Come on, Helen. Let's have a cup of coffee."

Florence later related to me what had happened when she found her in the Mall. When Florence spotted my Mother, she began waving and calling her name. My Mother spotted Florence and walked up to her. "Oh, Helen," she said, "I'm so glad I found you. I forgot where we were supposed to meet everyone." Florence, in her wisdom, simply said, "Oh, the meeting place has been changed. Everyone's waiting at home for you." My Mother said, "Oh, good. Then let's go."

If you have followed the chain of events here, you will realize what this story has told you. By the time my Mother got to the Mall, she forgot why she was going there. The event, in her mind, had changed to something else. Florence, as I said, in her wisdom, did not reprimand or panic my Mother with her actions, even though Florence was as close to hysteria as I was. She simply "went with the flow" and quietly brought her home.

Again, there are many, many stories that I could relate not only about my Mother, but many other folks who have experienced these types of situations. Wandering is a common behavior for people with Alzheimer's or a related disorder. Understanding why they do it is not the essential concern here. The mere fact that the possibility exists is where your major efforts need to be brought into play. It's not enough to simply "keep an eye out" for them or to try and monitor their actions around the house or on a daily basis. You need to take positive, direct action to try and prevent it from happening at all. God forbid, you should be one of those people who loses a parent or loved one, and they are never found or are found dead. Not a pretty picture, but we are dealing with a special type of reality here. Prevention is the key.

How, you say? There are several things you can do. First and foremost, as I mentioned in an earlier chapter, the Alzheimer's Association has what they call the Safe Return Program. It provides a safety net for the memory impaired and is the first and only nationwide community-based program to enable police, community agencies, hospitals and private citizens to help identify and assist in the safe return of Alzheimer's victims. Knowledge of the Safe Return Program is becoming widespread. It is no longer just an aid for doctors, hospitals, or police officials. Private citizens are becoming more and more aware of the Safe Return Program and the impact it can have on a person's well being and what it can mean to the families of the afflicted and lost. It is a very simple process.

First, call the national headquarters of the Alzheimer's Association located in Chicago, Illinois. Their toll-free number is 1-800-272-3900. Ask them to send you an application for registration in the program. When you receive it, fill it out along with a $25.00 registration fee. A pittance compared to what your losses might be.

The Safe Return Program provides registrants with an identity bracelet or necklace (that cannot be removed without sufficient assistance), clothing labels, and wallet ID cards. They are then registered in a *national database* connected to a network of law enforcement agencies. If the individual roams, a national 1-800 number can be located on the bracelet or necklace. A phone call is made to that national 1-800 number giving the individual identification number, also on the bracelet, to the person on the database line. They punch in that ID number and are able to come up with the lost individual's name, address, phone number, next of kin and their work and home numbers. Thus, the lost individual is re-connected with their families and caregivers.

Another method you can use to discourage roaming altogether is to put special locks on your doors. Because my Mother is such a wee thing, we were able to put simple slide locks way up on top of our doors that lead to the outside. We also have one on the basement door and another on the door leading out to the garage. She was never able to reach these locks and probably never noticed them. But this prevented her from opening any door and slipping outside. She did try to do this a couple of times before we put the locks on and we were able to catch her before she left the yard, but those few instances were enough to reinforce our thoughts of putting on those locks. Be careful with these locks. If you put locks that require keys, make sure you know where they are at all times and make sure you yourself can easily lock and unlock the device. There have been situations where a fire was started on the inside of the house, and because there were upper locks with padlocks that required keys, it nearly became a catastrophe for the entire family.

Do not think that this is an area that you need not concern yourself with. You might think in the back of your mind that your particular situation might be different and your loved one is not likely to roam. Nothing could be farther from the truth. I know of absolutely no cases to date where this has not become a problem. It is almost a universal behavior with all Alzheimer's victims, so prepare yourself early on and expect the unexpected.

Chapter 12

" . . . the most terrifying experience . . ."

Sundowning

This is yet another part of your experience which, I know, is completely foreign to you and is a rather strange phenomena. It is called sundowning. It usually begins to occur sometime in the late afternoon between the hours of 3:00 p.m. and 5:00 p.m. Again, I'm not sure exactly why it occurs, I can only voice my laymen's opinion but I would be willing to bet that I'm not too far off. Common sense is truly a magnificent trait. My common sense has kicked in more than once in my situation and has served me well in all instances.

All of us experience a sense of mental and physical fatigue towards the end of the day. It is the same with our poor victims. But these folks have been dealing with a barrel of scrambled mental conceptions and hallucinations for an entire day. Loss of memory, loss of independence, loss of self. Fear of discovery, fear of loss, fear of knowing that "something is not right." By the end of the day, the anxiety level is sky high.

This also is the time of day where the desire to roam may reach its peak. And the desire to do a lot of things may reach its peak. My Mother started on emptying drawers and closets during this time. She attempted to start laundry on several occasions right around 5:00. Any number of problems can arise during this period and you need to have alternative solutions. They may not be permanent solutions or may not be solutions at all but simply diversions. Either way you call it, it has to be something other than what they are focused to do at that moment if their activity appears that it may be destructive or disruptive.

I found several alternatives for my Mother and there is another key factor here in finding these alternatives. You may have to focus in on that particular individual's interests or hobbies. Possibly a life-long habit. For my Mother, I used to keep a pile of towels and washcloths in the laundry room in a basket just waiting for her. I would sit her down and give her this basket of laundry to fold over and over again. She would finish in about one half hour and I would take it into the laundry room and unfold it quickly and put it back in the basket. About five minutes later, bring the whole basket out for her to fold again. It worked wonderfully.

Shuffling cards and playing solitaire works in some instances. Crayons and coloring books.

Puzzles. Winding skeins of yarn into balls. Writing a grocery list. Cutting various holiday cut-outs out of colored construction paper. My Mother was an amateur painter so colored pencils and drawing paper kept her busy for long, long periods of time. When you put your mind to it, you can come up with a myriad of ideas.

Another good soother is music. My Mother loved to listen to old tunes from the 30's and the 40's. We put on a few tapes like Lawrence Welk, Glenn Miller, Jimmy Dorsey, and she would go to town. She danced all over the house for hours. Some people get relaxed with classical music or sometimes even New Age music. I knew one fellow who would sit for hours listening to Dixieland Jazz. The important thing is to find whatever your particular loved one may enjoy or more importantly, what they enjoyed doing in the past.

Here is another area where you need to dig deep in the recesses of your soul and remember that your love and your compassion for this afflicted soul is what is going to keep them from going over the edge. It is also, I might add, going to keep you from going over the edge. These can be extraordinarily trying times and you are going to go through this every single day. Another case where you need to expect the unexpected and prepare for the possibilities to stay ahead of this dastardly game. You'll never outsmart the affliction, but you can cleverly be on guard at every corner.

Chapter 13

" . . . the few moments of spontaneous levity . . . "

Spirit

It's funny how Spirit just naturally comes into play every couple of chapters. And here we are again, repeating it. But it's always been said that repetition is the key to success. Practice makes perfect.

But this chapter on Spirit is a bit different. This time we need to talk about the Spirit of our poor, waning loved ones whose Spirit just keeps kicking and keeps rearing its delightful but intruding head every inch of the way, sometimes creating havoc for all those around. This is probably where your love and your patience and your understanding are going to have the greatest test of all.

I have always said throughout this book that it is vitally necessary that you DO NOT reprimand, scold or even try to correct mistakes that are made by our loved ones. And this is the reason. It is only the survival of their own Spirit that keeps driving them.

As we discussed, there is a lifetime of habitual behavior imprisoned in their souls. There is a lifetime of *duty* and *responsibility* engrained in their existence. There is a lifetime of diversified activity that continues to bounce around in their being, screaming for acknowledgment and release. All for the sole purpose of relieving their anxiety and mental confusion.

You can take away certain functions and capabilities from any individual. You can take a long list of things that exist within any individual. But you can never completely take away their Spirit for survival. Even a drowning man, as he sinks to the bottom of the ocean, is still thinking of how he can survive.

All Spirit that exists in all living things is the mightiest of power. It will keep them searching for those lost children. It will keep them moving around the house in a hundred different directions. It will keep them doing all sorts of things that are going to frustrate the hell out of you. But remember in your heart, when you feel that you are at your wit's end, it is their Spirit that is fighting. Fighting for survival and a normal state of mind. Do not deny them that right to fight for survival by reprimanding and scolding.

Again, you have to learn to go with the flow. And the same goes for any and all persons who are going to have any interaction with the stricken individual. They need to understand this concept and they need to accept it in their hearts.

I have friends whose stricken fathers still try to get out to go to work. That was their duty and responsibility. Others will tell their children that Mabel is coming to get them for Bridge. That was an activity that went on for many years. Others will try to get out or search the house for cigarettes. That is habitual behavior. But behind all of it, is the Spirit fighting. Fighting to make everything okay. Fighting to prove to them that everything is okay.

I don't honestly know if allowing the Spirit to continue to exist is right or wrong. All I can tell you, again, is what I experienced and what I went through. And my gut extinct is to let it flow for as long as it needs to. This is the same Spirit we talked about in the other chapter. The God-given one that rises to the occasion for <u>you</u> when you least expect it, the Spirit that bleeds compassion and love when you least expect it. It is <u>your</u> power and it is yours to keep. It is not our job or our right to try and take it away from someone else.

After many years battling with this disease, I still went out on the patio with my Mother on occasion and shared a cigarette and a cocktail with her. I spoke to our physician about smoking and drinking alcohol. He simply said, "This is all they have left. Taking it away from them isn't going to save their life." But to my Mother, this was enforcing her Spirit and giving her a connection to a former self. Rest assured, both old habits were closely monitored, but enjoying a cigarette and a cocktail once in a while gave her a sense of normalcy and acceptance. She knew that I knew that "something was not right." But I know she appreciated the fact that I didn't let it interfere with our connection as Mother and Daughter and our desire to treat ourselves to a cigarette and a cocktail out on the patio.

Time certainly doesn't make things any better. But remembering <u>their</u> Spirit during this time of tragic lessening makes an enormous difference in how you manage and how they manage.

But, the most important thing of all to remember is this. Respect their Spirit at all times. When it is time and your loved one must leave, their Spirit may linger awhile to help you through, and perhaps bestow good things upon you for respecting and remembering. That's just how they are.

Chapter 14

" . . . your own survival as a caregiver. "

Outside Help

Yes, your own survival as a caregiver. This is a vitally important factor in this whole process and should never be swept under the rug for reasons of shame, guilt, expense or any such other excuse you think you might make. In practically every other facet of our life, we consider outside help. We hire cleaning ladies. We call painters to paint the house. We hire babysitters to give us some time to ourselves. We call on hundreds of outside, skilled workers to perform any number of tasks for us simply because we are possibly overbooked, overworked or overextended. During this time of transition, you will be all of the above and looking to outside help is only a sensible and practical avenue.

FAMILY AND FRIENDS

I mentioned very early on some suggestions that you might consider, starting with family and friends. If you have done your due diligence in the early stages, you will have informed all family and friends of your oncoming situation and prepared everyone for all the stages that lie before you. During your conversations, do not be afraid to mention that you will probably be needing some help as time goes on, and any time that they can spare will be greatly appreciated. You might even be able to look to your closer family members for some regular scheduling alternatives. If you have an extended family, you might be one of the lucky ones who will be able to look to those family members for continual assistance several times a week, or possibly every day.

You are going to need help with everything from meal preparation to grocery shopping to doctor's appointments. Realistically, one person certainly is able to do all those things, but when you have someone who cannot be left alone and as time goes on, will not be physically able to freely or easily move about without some kind of assistance, you will not be able to take them with you every time you go out the door to tend to business. They simply will not be physically able to travel around with you. You will have to rely on other people to either assist you with your errands, or to stay with your loved one while you tend to outside duties.

Along with family and friends, there are several places you can go for suggestions or possible assistance. I also stated earlier that you will find many inroads to where you can go for help, but you will also find, along the way, the help that you will desperately need will simply not be available to you. This is where we encounter the double-edged sword and this is where I have huge criticisms with regard to our healthcare system, or perhaps I should say, the lack of our healthcare system. But we will get to that later. For now, let's just concentrate on the positive and see where we can direct you.

ALZHEIMER'S ASSOCIATION

I have also mentioned earlier the Alzheimer's Association. This is a national organization that is dedicated to aiding families in crisis and providing information to all members with regard to research, healthcare reform, pharmaceutical advances for Alzheimer's, support groups, home care assistance, and any number of areas that might assist a family in need of help who has suddenly become burdened with this deadly disease. It is comprised of members who have been through or who are going through the devastation of Alzheimer's with a loved one. Their national headquarters is in Chicago, Illinois and you can call their office at 1-800-272-3900 to find out the closest chapter to your area. The support groups are especially helpful and meaningful. At these meetings, you are able to interact with people who are going through the same things that you are experiencing and you can share problems, information and even phone numbers. A lot of helpful information is transferred and gained at these meetings.

CAREGIVER AGENCIES

There are also outside caregiver or companion agencies that offer assistance for elder care and some of these agencies specialize in care for Alzheimer's patients. They run the gamut from hourly care a few times a week all the way to full-time, live-in care. They can be rather expensive, and unfortunately, the average household is not equipped to handle a price tag of $600 to $700 to $800 a week for a live-in. The average runs about $18.00 per hour for a minimum of an 8 hour day. That's $144.00 per day multiplied by 5 days, and you get $720.00 per week. Pretty pricey. Of course, there certainly are some folks who are well equipped to handle these kinds of expenses. God bless them if they can afford it. I just don't happen to run in those circles! But, perhaps, at least once or twice a week might be workable.

CHURCH GROUPS

Another alternative is to contact your local church groups. If you are a regular member of any church in your area, you can get in touch with your board or council members and see if there is some kind of assistance group within your church council. There may be a strong volunteer group that you may not be aware of and if there isn't, you might be the one to start it and get the embers glowing to institute a program like this within your church. There are probably many, many retired people who might like to make a little extra money. I heard of one church who has a volunteer group of over 100 retired people from the congregation. They usually are willing to do the work for nothing, but the norm is to give them at least $5.00 an hour for their time. This sounded like a win-win situation to me and everybody was happy and everybody was helped. It doesn't hurt to make the phone call. If nothing is available there, you will probably get other suggestions or even phone numbers from your contacts to further your quest.

DAY CARE FACILITIES

Recently, there has been a great improvement in the number of day care facilities available for the elderly. It seems that every week a new one pops up in our area. These are simply day care centers where you can take your loved one early in the morning and pick them up later in the afternoon. Just as they run the day care centers for children, these facilities are well-equipped to handle all types of Alzheimer's patients. The fees are usually quite reasonable and you can use the facilities for one day or two or for the entire week if you need it. These facilities are usually connected with one of your local hospitals. Be aware, however, that if your loved one is infirm or immobile, in all likelihood, they will not be able to participate or be accepted into one of these facilities.

Early on, I was able to take my Mother to one of these facilities. Depending on the size, they have a full-trained staff of 4 or 5 individuals to care for and entertain the patients. They have arts and crafts, sing-a-longs, flower arranging, story-telling, piano players, animal groups that come in, any number of varied activities throughout each day to keep them busy and fulfilled. My Mother's group even had a Prom one day where they had records for dancing and punch and a good time was had by all. I volunteered that day to assist with the festivities and still have pictures. I keep them close at hand to remind me of those few precious moments I was still able to have with my Mother. Even though she was ill and we both knew it, we still danced, pranced, and laughed like hell. It was another "connection" for her and a wonderful experience for me. You should be able to find the locations of these facilities by looking in the phone book or contacting your local area hospitals. Also, the Alzheimer's Association should have a good handle of what is available in your area. Word of mouth is another good way to get information, so dig around your neighborhood or your friends and find out what's going on in your community. There's probably a lot more activity in this area than you ever thought.

NURSING HOMES

I have tried to avoid this subject through this entire book because my mission here is to give you information and guidance on how to specifically care for your loved one in the home. My personal choice was to keep my Mother at home with me for the rest of her living days. And I will keep to that decision no matter what. I will interject here, not my personal opinion, but my personal feelings on the whole nursing home scenario. I don't like them. I don't trust them. And I surely wouldn't want to be in one. There. So sue me.

Our family physician is currently on the board of three nursing homes in our area. He has told me, with heavy heart, some of his experiences from dealing with these homes. He works an 80 hour week between his practice and keeping these nursing homes on their toes. Unfortunately, he has told me, as good as some of them try to be, their existence depends entirely on their financial success or failure. And most of them are always bordering on the financial edge. He also told me that with the kind of care that my Mother gets at home, I would never be happy with <u>any</u> nursing home care for her. We have all heard of the horrific stories of abuse and neglect that can go on in these homes, and because of that, I harbor a profound fear of them. But even setting the worst aside, just the emotional aspects of dealing with the idea is almost incomprehensible to me. I have seen the terror in my Mother's eyes when she looks across the street and sees the bank, thinking it's a nursing home. I have to hold her and caress her and gently reinforce in her that she is home with me, and no one will ever take her away from me. And that I will never leave her. As she calms, her body becomes less rigid, her breathing slows, and her eyes just slowly blink to tell me she believes me, and that she believes IN me. And we rock back and forth while I hold her in my arms. I would not sleep nights thinking of my Mother lying in bed asking God why I abandoned her.

I understand that many folks feel that they have no alternative. But I also know that many people simply don't want to be bothered because it might be too much work or inconvenience. I heard of a story about a gentlemen who was a college professor and was on some kind of lecture circuit. In the meantime, his stricken Mother was at home with full-time care. He made it his business to get home to her, no matter where he was in the country, every three to four days. After several weeks of exhaustive travel, one of his colleagues said to him, "Why don't you put her in a nursing home? She wouldn't know the difference. She doesn't even know who you are." He simply answered, "But I know who she is." And therein is the full tale.

My Mother cleaned and nurtured my scraped knees and elbows, came to every dance recital, baked my favorite cookies, knit me sweaters, made prom dresses, and held my hand while I cried my eyes out the first day I got my period. And this is the woman that I'm going to conveniently sweep off to a nursing home because it's more convenient for me?!? So you see, I have extraordinarily strong feelings on this issue. However, again, I do understand that there may truly be instances where a nursing home may be in the best interest of the entire family. Particularly if there are many young children and the possibly of constant disruption of routine could be critical to their upbringing.

But if you feel that this is the best alternative for you and your family there is a long list of things to consider when choosing a home for your loved one. A few are: location, your ability to communicate with the staff, amount of staff available or the ratio of staff to patients, medical services on hand, restraint policies, food services, fire safety, payment considerations, Medicare and Medicaid possibilities and eligibility, etc. Always visit any considered home more than once and without announcement. Talk to the residents. And by all means, review your contract before signing and possibly let your attorney review it for you. Do not sign ANYTHING without first being given the opportunity to take it home and review it completely. The U.S. Department of Health and Human Services puts out a wonderful booklet that gives you all sorts of guidelines when choosing a nursing home.

In conclusion on this subject, I have just two things to say. Do extensive, and I mean extensive, research on your choice of facilities. And the other is, I hope you can find one for less than $4,000 a month! (To be discussed in a later chapter.)

ADVERTISE

Another way that people have found help, is simply through the want-ads of your local newspaper. Determine what you can afford, what amount of time you may need someone, and go from there. If you place an ad, you might be surprised at what you find. But, again, be smart in your search and ask for, get, and check references. And do extensive research on the individual, i.e., police record, possible credit check, job history. Credit and job check could be an indication as to the degree of an individual's sense of responsibility.

VISITING DOCTOR

This is one of the blessings that I've found to be almost a found miracle of the century. We all know that house-calls from physicians are pretty much a thing of the past. However, there is a new phenomena happening around the country and that is the visiting doctor for elder care. I have found one and I believe this man to be next to sainthood. He has become our family physician and if he ever moves to another state, I believe we will move with him.

As the victim's mobility begins to decline, it will become more and more difficult to get the individual out of the house for the much needed medical review on a regular basis. I had a doctor for my Mother who was prescribing some medicine for her. It was a simple anti-anxiety prescription. I called his office one day to ask him to call the pharmacy for a refill on the prescription. He refused to do so and asked that my Mother come in for a check-up. At this point, my Mother could barely move her little legs from her bed to her wheelchair to get to the bathroom. Every movement had become and still is a major, major struggle for her and those of us who are assisting her. Asking my Mother to get to the doctor's office was like asking a six year old child to carry eight pieces of luggage through an airport. Virtually impossible. Needless to say, I fired that physician and began a search for a new and more compassionate man who understood the difficult situation I was in. And, with my faith in mankind and my faith in life itself, I found him!

He comes to the house every 90 to 120 days to do a routine check on my Mother and her physical health. He tells me that he can't believe the condition she is in for the condition she is in. He believes she is doing so well physically because of her emotional balance and the balance of life and love that we continue to create around her. Now mind you, she is in very bad shape with regard to the Alzheimer's situation. She can no longer walk, talk, feed herself, get herself to the bathroom, bathe herself, etc. But her heart and her lungs and her blood are healthy, healthy, healthy.

I believe that when people are grossly unhappy, i.e., nursing home situations, they can will themselves to die. And you ask any nursing home employee and they will tell you the same thing. But in my Mother's situation, she is hanging on because she is home. She is loved and nurtured on a daily basis and she gets magnificent care. Her needs are met on a 24-hour basis, both physical and emotional. And as I have stressed throughout this book, the emotional part is what is so vitally important for their well-being and their comfort zone. I believe my Mother, even in the condition she is in, has no desire to leave this life just yet. I believe she understands somewhat that she is in a very bad situation where her mental health is concerned, but she is very comfortable with her surroundings and suffers nothing in that respect.

But even though my Mother's mental health is deteriorating on a daily basis, I still feel a moral and compassionate obligation to see to it that her physical health is reviewed regularly. And these visiting doctors are a God send. But I must warn you. There are organizations or agencies out there that will advertise home-care or visiting doctor agencies that group together and send doctors to your home for the alleged health visitation. I had one experience with one of these visiting doctor agencies and promptly removed them from my list after the first visit. After I made an appointment and waited two and one-half hours for this doctor to show up for his scheduled visit, he spent all of ten minutes with my Mother and charged Medicare $240.00. I had asked him to do a blood check and a heart check and he came prepared with nothing and said we needed to schedule another visit with him. And, of course, this would cost an additional $240.00. Oh, and the blood and heart tests would be extra. I was so angry with this set-up, I began to do some investigating. I found that this particular doctor who was hired by this doctors' agency, was a tattoo removal specialist and had absolutely no credentials or experience working with the elderly or Alzheimer's. So my point is, just because they call themselves doctors, doesn't necessarily mean that they know what they're doing in this particular field.

As in any case when you hiring on an individual to do any work for you, check references, background, experience, etc. Too many people take for gospel everything that any doctor (or lawyer, for that matter) says without question simply because they call themselves doctors or lawyers. Trust me, if there are bad painters or bad mechanics or bad anything, there are bad doctors and lawyers. Don't get me wrong. I know there are many, many good and even great doctors and lawyers out there. But keep yourself protected from the not-so-great ones by doing your due diligence. As a consumer, or even more simply, as a human being, you have the right to question and even investigate, so don't be afraid to ask for and expect references or credentials. And make sure you get them.

The best thing to do is to check with other family members or friends, or even members of the Alzheimer's Association for names and numbers of visiting doctors. Here again, you may be surprised at what you find.

ADULT FOSTER CARE

There is yet another alternative to either part-time or full-time outside help. There are various facilities around the country that offer a more communal or family atmosphere in terms of care and surroundings. These are actually much smaller group homes, probably individual family-type situations, that take in only a minimal number of people to live in their home either on a full-time or day-care basis. The situation offers a closer knit environment offering activities throughout the day, or simply just a quiet day of movies or television. Meals, of course, are included as is any physical or hygiene assistance. The cost of these facilities is much more reasonable ranging from around $6,000 to $24,000 a year depending on the amount of time needed in the facility. But here, again, you must remember to do your due diligence and get references and/or recommendations from the outside. I would hate to think that I am leaving my loved one somewhere thinking their needs are being fully cared for only to find out that there is either abuse or neglect involved. Just as there are problems for parents and their children in their day-care situations, there are the same concerns for our incapacitated elderly. For more out-of-home care options, you can write to Family Caregiver Alliance, 690 Market Street, Suite 600, San Francisco, California, 94104 or visit their website at www.caregiver.com. You can also contact the American Association of Retired Persons (AARP) at 601 E St., N.W., Washington, D.C. 20049 or visit www.aarp.org.

LIVE-IN CAREGIVERS

This is probably my most favorite subject to discuss. More and more people are learning the ropes of having full-time live-in caregivers and the advantages of doing so. Had I not had a full-time live-in, I doubt seriously that I would have maintained my sanity over the last 14 years. Aside from the errands and family business needs mentioned earlier, there is a question of your own mental health while caring for the victims. Now, I don't mean to say that you will go completely crazy, or have a breakdown, or any such thing. But I will say this. You could possibly come damn close. The strain of 24 hour, 7 day a week care, is something I never considered. And when it begins to creep up on you, if you're lucky, you will recognize that there is a gray cloud that seems to hover over you. At the first sign of recognition, DO SOMETHING! I cannot tell you how devastating the repercussions can be if you don't. If you ignore your first signs of overwork and overload, a depression begins to settle in that will knock you for a loop. You won't even know what's happening until it may be too late. Your attitude begins to change, your habits begin to change, and sometimes, even your walk and your talk begin to change. These are danger signals.

A few people have mentioned to me that caring for an Alzheimer's victim is like caring for a child. It's worse. A child continues to grow and learn and each day can do more and more for himself. In our situation, the complete opposite happens. The victim begins to forget how to do everything from buttoning a shirt to going to the bathroom, or even how to lift a fork and put it to their mouth. Each day the victims can do less and less for themselves. And each day, it is your job to do more and more, no matter how frustrated or tired you become. You can sink into a deep, deep depression and before you know it, you are almost as helpless as your victim. That is why seeking outside help and perhaps getting a live-in, is in the best interest of all concerned.

Expenses, you say. In the last 14 years, I have learned many, many ways to get around a huge expense of having a live-in. First, I don't go to the agencies. As mentioned earlier, the expense of agencies is almost out of reach for most of us. However, going private, or seeking your own assistance, can be well within your means. I have had my own experiences and heard a number of stories on how folks have connected and were able to find good, caring and loving people to care for their loved ones. It just takes a little imagination and determination, but there are several ways to find people.

First, try your local churches. It doesn't have to be your specific denomination, so get the phone book out and start calling. I mentioned earlier about the volunteer groups, but sometimes there are other groups within that same church that do other types of activities. I know there are several Polish, Mexican, Greek, etc. churches in the Chicago area that are continually bringing folks here for proposed residency. While the families love the idea of having their relatives come here, at times the financial burden does not make that possible, not to mention the lack of sufficient space to take another individual into their home. But if there was another alternative for their out-of-country relative, the families would be thrilled to bring them. That's where you come in. You can call some of these churches and leave your name and number. There may already be someone in the wings who is waiting to find some place to live and to make a little money. There is, of course, the issue of paying Social Security taxes. You will need to check with your local Social Security office to get details and paperwork. Your helper also must need a work permit in order to work for you. These issues can get kind of tricky, but with a little perseverance, you can muddle through the details and get things in order. It's not that difficult.

I have heard many, many stories of how families were able to bring on board someone from this type of situation. They were thrilled to have their room and board and sometimes they will work for as little as $200 a week to start. This is very, very inexpensive help and well worth the effort and time. Most of these folks have turned out to be most reliable and very caring and loving in their responsibilities with the elder care. It will be up to you to set your guidelines with them on just how much you want them to do and the exact type of care you want your loved one to have. Sometimes language can be a barrier, but only in the beginning. The transfer of languages is a most rewarding experience for both yourself and your caregiver. They are learning English and you are learning a second language, something you never thought you would do.

Another alternative might be your own family if you still have relatives in other countries. This was my situation. I had a distant cousin in Poland who became a widow at age 60. There are no jobs to speak of in Poland and money is very scarce as is food and other necessities of life. Because she could not afford to keep her home, it was necessary for her to move in with a daughter. Now there were five mouths to feed instead of four and barely a space for her to sleep. I made a deal with her. She was able to get a visa to come here, I paid her ticket and she now lives with me full-time and helps me take care of my Mother. This care is in exchange for her room and board. When she goes out or goes to visit other friends or some of our other relatives, I always see that she has $50 or $100 in her pocket so she is not penniless when she goes out the door. This is a small price to pay for her tender love and care and continual availability. And she is always most grateful for anything I do for her. I love her dearly and we are now on our way to getting citizenship for her.

When my Mother passes, my cousin will stay with me and perhaps she can assist some other family who may need a loving caregiver for their stricken loved one. These helpers are truly "angels of mercy" and have given me the ability to spend quality time with my Mother. I am able to sit with her and just talk, or sing, or just stroke her frightened little head and try to make things " all better" for her. We watch TV and we color in coloring books and do all sorts of activities. And my time with her is not spent feeding, bathing, cleaning, and getting stressed out. My time with her is spent loving her and letting her know that I'm here for her. My stress level is practically nil and my communication with her is soft, gentle and reminiscent of my childhood when my Mother would speak softly to me, hug me, hold me, and tell me she loved me and that everything is okay. Now it's my turn.

Whether it's a parent, a spouse, an aunt, an uncle, a grandparent or even a friend. When someone is embarking on this terror-filled journey, they need to hear that they are loved a thousand times a day. Perhaps, now, it's your turn to offer those words with as much warmth and kindness and compassion that you can give. Having an "angel of mercy" gives you the opportunity to be relatively stress free, and lets you open your gates to let your love flow evenly, regularly and honestly. Do that for your loved one and do that for yourself.

Chapter 15

"... careful planning and preparation ..."

Financial and Legal

Throughout this book, I have stressed how careful planning and preparation plays an important role in your survival as a caregiver in the areas of actual physical caregiving. We now journey into an area that becomes distasteful to most and can develop into a heart wrenching process for yourself and your family unless you open your minds and hearts. If you go into your planning process with an open mind, you will forge forward with all the necessary information needed for a successful survival plan for you, your loved one, and your family. If you go into the planning process with an open heart, you will not only do justice to the needs of yourself and your family, but you will do justice to the needs and concerns of your loved one. Yes, they will have needs. But, they also have concerns about their future, their family and everything else that goes along with it including their money, their house, their personal possessions, their prized mementos.

This is probably the most difficult area because there are decisions that need to be made that may not be to your liking or to the satisfaction of certain members of your family. Further, there are issues that will need to be confronted early on that you or your loved one or members of your family are going to feel uneasy about discussing and a typical reaction would be "Oh, let's not talk about that now." Unfortunately, NOW is the best time to talk about it and NOW is the absolute time to talk about it.

If you think about it, most people are already half way there in their "life or death" preparations, i.e., wills, living wills, cemetery plots, trusts, etc. All these things are items that are carefully thought out and planned in advance of any individual's demise. When you discover that you have an advancing army in the guise of continued deterioration of the mind and body, it only makes sense to begin planning for both your physical needs and your financial and legal needs as well. In fact, it would behoove all of us to develop these types of plans right along with our wills and trusts, etc., because one never knows when these vicious diseases will strike. And the trauma of the affliction is difficult enough to deal with without having the extra burden of planning for survival at the last minute.

I know many people today who are doing just that. And, I must say, that my parents prepared themselves reasonably well for what the future may have held long before my Mother was stricken. This preparation made life much simpler for me when I had to take over my Mother's care and also, when my Father passed away, the transition of all properties and assets was an easy one. But let's start at the beginning and work our way through the maze of legal and financial issues with as much practicality as we can muster and try to divorce ourselves from the emotions that will try to overcome us in the process.

PRE-PLANNED FACILITY CARE

Again, this may not be the most pleasant of tasks, but may be one of, if not the biggest, issue that you will have to deal with in your pre-planning. There are many folks today who are visiting and pre-registering for facility care long before any signs appear or at the very, very earliest of detection.

I know I stated earlier my negative feelings about nursing homes or nursing facilities. Please be assured that this is only a personal opinion and I am certainly not trying to cast aspersions on the industry as a whole or negate any thoughts of contemplating nursing facilities. In my personal situation, I had to deal with my Mother's terror of nursing homes. And I suppose that this may have come from her early experiences when dealing with her grandmother and the types of facility care that was available back in the 20's and 30's.

Today, there are many, many types of nursing or assisted living facilities that range anywhere from private one or two bedroom units in an assisted living complex or development to full range multiple unit nursing care facilities. You may be able to start with an assisted living situation and as time goes on, progress into a full nursing facility. The point is, pre-planning is the key.

There are many people who are adamant about not being a "burden" to their families and their loved ones and do not want anyone in their family to be saddled with the responsibility of their full-time care in the event of the onslaught of a devastating disease like Alzheimer's. They make this decision early on, investigate their possibilities, and demand that their families adhere to their requests by placing them in a facility when they feel the time is right. This is perfectly acceptable as a solution. But, unfortunately, the expense can be extraordinary and usually pre-arrangement requires some form of pre-payment or some pledge of possessions, property or financial assets. Of course, the individuals who are choosing this avenue, certainly have the right to pledge anything they own. But at times, this is where the dissatisfaction of other family members may come into play. This is where problems may occur due to family members who think they should have a "piece of the family pie" and pledging everything to an outside facility will not be to their liking. They seem to forget that the "family pie" was not theirs to begin with, and certainly they should have no say in how it is deemed for use by the "owners." On the other hand, if there is a question of inheritance, most parents do, in fact, want the bulk of their estate to go to their children and grandchildren. So, you see, the decision-making can be quite complex and this is where pre-planning is most important.

At any rate, this type of pre-planning and pre-registering is more and more becoming a widely used avenue for seniors in their choices for their future.

ASSESSING YOUR FINANCES

One of the first things you need to do is to sit down and make lists of your current financial standing and resources. If you are a spouse of the afflicted individual, you will need to consider things such as current income, limited income after retirement, property, stock holdings, anything and everything that you hold, own or have investment in that may be affected. You will also have to take into consideration the possibility of lost income if your spouse has been working. If you are a child or relative, you need to make this list on behalf of the afflicted individual to find out what their resources are in order to make plans for their financial future and potential care.

Then, of course, you will need to make a list of current and potential expenses including housing, outside help, medical expenses, food, and possible nursing home expenses. If you intend to keep the impaired individual at home with you, you may think that there will be no additional expenses. How wrong you are! You absolutely must remember what I wrote earlier. You have to have additional help for yourself in this journey. There is no possible way that you will be able to handle every hour of every day of every week, etc., totally and completely on your own! It is imperative that you have some kind of respite care available to you on a regular basis. You may have your friends or other relatives on a list, or even on a schedule. Things come up, and sometimes these persons are not going to be available to you on their regularly scheduled day or days. But you, as the primary caregiver, must have your time to yourself. That's why it's necessary to have other outside alternatives for that help, even if you have to pay for it.

After you have completed all these lists and weighed each one against the other, you will, more than likely, find yourself coming up short. Search for other resources. Check your insurance policies and see what is available to you for home care. Again, check volunteer groups from churches or senior community groups. Get involved with your local Alzheimer's Association chapters and get all the info you can. This is where the realization of what lies before you is going to hit home.

LONG-TERM CARE INSURANCE

Another thing to consider is checking into long-term care insurance. This will probably do you no good when you are at the front gate of your potential journey. But I feel the need to, at least, propose and briefly discuss this subject in case you are one of those persons who is reading this book merely for information even if you currently do not have this problem confronting you. And perhaps you can just pass this on to someone else. Long-term care insurance is probably one of the best things we've got going for us in the insurance game. But it's not cheap. When the time comes when you might have to put this insurance into play, all you do is make a phone call and your needs are met on a continuing basis. It covers everything from a visiting nurse once a week and medical appliances all the way to full-time home care or nursing home care. It is not a bad idea to look into long-term care. Like I said, it isn't cheap but in the long run, it may be your best avenue.

MEDICARE AND MEDICAID

Medicare and Medicaid are always areas that you need to look into. However, be very careful in your plans to rely on this avenue. I remember in

1994 a law was passed that enabled any government welfare agency to file a claim for reimbursement against a deceased client or surviving spouse's estate. In other words, if you found it necessary to turn to Medicare or Medicaid for assistance in any type of nursing home care, they can place a lien on the deceased client's estate or the surviving spouse's estate. This means that for every penny that was spent by Medicare for the care of your loved one in a nursing home, they can reimburse themselves from your estate, thereby depleting any inheritance that you had marked for your children by that amount. As horrific as these practices sound, I am simply trying to make you aware of every nook and cranny that you need to look into and need to consider, or, on the negative side, NOT consider.

There is something called PACE (Program of All-Inclusive Care for the Elderly) and S/HMO (Social Health Maintenance Organizations) that are connected to Medicare and Medicaid that offer a little more. But these programs are not available in all states and you need to contact your local Medicare and Medicaid service agency to find out if your state has these programs available.

Medicare and Medicaid is absolutely available for seniors and their continuing health situations. However, there are great restrictions on types of care and eligibility that make it nearly impossible to allow you to be a participant in any nursing home payment program. These programs will not pay for any in-home assistance on a full-time basis, only visiting nursing care after a hospital stay. If you are eligible for full-time nursing home financial assistance, there are special government certified facilities that you must use and you have a limited choice of these facilities. Eligibility in itself can be a nightmare. The bulk of your estate must be "spent down" or "gifted" to your children several years prior to application as you are allowed minimal financial holdings in order to be eligible for Medicare assistance. Ten years ago, my Father began "gifting" me on an annual basis with certain sums of money that he transferred from his estate to me. There is also a restriction of how much can be transferred or "gifted" annually. By the time my parents became my full-time responsibility, I had well over $100,000 that had been legally "gifted" and transferred over to me. I am an only child and most honorable, if I do say so myself. So for those ten years, I did not so much as touch one penny of that money as it was really not mine to touch. The money was finally utilized as a down payment on a rather large home that my Father requested we build. This was for the sole purpose of having a space large enough for them when the time would come when my husband and I needed to take over full-time care for both my Mother and my Father. Eventually, it did become necessary for both of them to move in permanently with us. Unfortunately, there are those individuals who may not be able to resist the temptation to dip into those funds. On the other hand, some seniors feel that their children are going to inherit it anyway, so, as my Father once told me, "What's the difference if you get it now or get it later." Again, this is yet another decision that you need to make that will not be an easy one.

OPTIONS

The problems are many. As you can see, there is not much help for us middle-class folks and most people spend a life-time working and squirreling away to the best of their ability only to have it claimed by outside forces in times of crisis.

Nursing home or in-home assistance restrictions and the change in the estate recovery laws is now forcing another avenue that seniors are considering as an option. And that option is divorce. By divorcing, the well spouse or surviving spouse is not responsible for any extraordinary hospital, medical or nursing home expenses should the afflicted individual need Medicare assisted nursing facility care. The divorce also allows the afflicted spouse to become eligible for government assistance without the necessity of a "spend down" if all assets have become the sole property of the well spouse. In other words, you don't have to gift, hide or get rid of your assets or income as your well spouse, or now, your ex-spouse will have complete control of all assets and income with the exception of pension or social security which would have to be signed over to the nursing facility anyway.

These negative options do not paint a pretty picture of the state of affairs for this country for our seniors. These types of negative options or negative planning devices are affecting the very structure of our families and family values. It is a sad state, indeed, when one reaches their "golden years" that they have to spend time planning on how to "circumvent the systems" in order to survive or simply try to hold on to what they have worked their entire lives to gain. But this is yet another chapter.

My main message here is to plan, plan, plan. Do it early enough while all persons are still competent and able to make intelligent decisions regarding their future and the futures of their loved ones.

Find yourself an attorney who specializes in estate planning and who has the experience of dealing with all the problems that can arise during situations like this. Ask your friends, ask your neighbors, get on the Internet, contact the Alzheimer's Association. Do whatever you have to do to get your affairs in order. Do not leave yourself wide open for disappointment and frustration.

There are hundreds of thousands of seniors in this country who are scrambling for financial and emotional assistance during this time of horrific crisis. I currently know three families who are right in the middle of this crisis and can't seem to pull themselves free from the daily chaos simply because they did not plan early enough, even though they knew this mysterious monster was slowly moving its way into their lives. They took no notice and made no plans. So, today, they are "scrambling" trying to take care of their afflicted loved ones, their own families and themselves. And trying to figure out how they are going to financially and emotionally survive, if at all.

"Careful planning and preparation" is the only way to survive. "Careful planning and preparation" is the only way to keep chaos and terror at bay, and the only way to keep your love flowing freely, unencumbered. Remember, this is our mission. This is our job.

Chapter 16

"... understand the scientific explanations ... "

Research and Medicine

Science and intellect can never, ever prepare you for what you are about to experience. The first signs appear to be easy enough to deal with. And you think that "this can't be so bad." Then, as time begins to creep along, those same insignificant signs go by the wayside only to be replaced by bigger and more noticeable ones. As each set of problems replaces itself with yet an even larger set of problems, your brain begins to scream for answers. Why? Why is this happening to us? What brings about this devastation? What can one do? Where does one go for answers? And then you ask why, again, only to arrive back at square one with no answers, no solutions, no place to go for a cure, no help on the horizon, even if only temporary.

Over the past decade or so, Alzheimer's has become a celebrity. A famous and well-known entity that has been brought out of the closet and paraded around the globe, lifting its head, snubbing its nose, as if to say, here! Here I am! Now what? As though we didn't have enough to worry about on this planet and enough problems to solve and enough diseases to cure.

Yes, it's been brought out of the closet, but rest assured, it has been around a long, long time. Victorian times called it senility as did the eras of the 30', 40's, and 50's. But as we sneaked our way into the 60's and 70's, we became a throw-away society and simply swept or neatly tucked our family "nuts" away somewhere, either in institutions or attics. But the 90's surprised us all. This disease lunged out and reared its ugly head loudly and clearly for all to hear. It forced the world to recognize it and forced mankind to dig deep into the depths of his understanding not only to search for a cause and a cure, but to search his own being for any thread of compassion, to look into the eyes of a victim and understand their fear and their terror and finally realize that "throwing them away" is not the answer.

What is this brain-wasting disease? To us "lay" folks, Alzheimer's has been stated as a "condition that results in loss of intellectual capacity and impairs both social and occupational functioning." Pretty simple. Pretty devastating. Scientifically, research has told us it is plaque on the brain. More specifically, scientists have identified an enzyme called beta-secretase which plays a key role in the buildup of abnormal plaques in the brain.

These plaques, from a protein called beta amyloid, destroy brain cells. Another enzyme, gamma-secretase, is thought to play a key role in abnormal build-up of the protein, beta amyloid. So the trick is to prevent the abnormal build-up of these particular enzymes. This is prevention. And believe it or not, there is already work being done to develop a vaccine for immunization against Alzheimer's. Unfortunately, we are told that it would be "premature" to give any timeline on completion of development. All research is in its infancy.

To this date, there is no cure for this murderous invader, but over the last several years, various medications have been developed that allegedly arrest the continued development of the disease. The key to any success in this type of treatment is to catch the symptoms early enough so treatment is constructive rather than destructive. If the disease goes unnoticed or worse, if those around the victim attempt to function in a state of denial for any length of time, the advancement of the disease may be at a point where arresting the further development may only prolong the inevitable and make continuing life at that level a torturous endeavor for all parties. This could be disastrous for both the caregiver and the victim in that somewhere about mid-point in the disease is usually the worst time for both.

The beginning of the disease is confusing and frightening, while the advanced stages are sad, but more quieting. The middle stages can be horrendous, volatile and the most difficult emotionally and physically. Prolonging the mid-stage will create hostility and frustration and break down the wall of protection and comfort that is so vital to the victim. It can cause those closest to the victim to walk away and seek refuge anyhow and anywhere, leaving the victim in a state of terror as they are pushed into nursing home arenas and left, they feel, abandoned by all those they love. However, if symptoms are recognized early enough, treatment can, in fact, arrest the disease and keep the victim in the beginning stages, which is not perfect, but certainly tolerable. As I stated, recognizing the symptoms or catching the signals is key to successful treatment. It is also key to successful planning.

Two of the drugs for early treatment are Cognex and Aricept. But confer with your physician on these drugs. Research is continual and there may be other types out there, but most of these drugs have side affects that are not particularly pleasant. There is also some dispute as to whether or not these drugs are effective at all. Apparently, research showed that there could be considerable improvement, but actual case histories, at times, showed differently. The actual success of these drugs may be on an individual basis only.

For years, a cure for Alzheimer's has always been an arm's reach away from researchers. Over the last few years, that gap has been shortened and scientists believe they may be on the brink of an important breakthrough in finding a cure - an absolute reversal of brain cell damage and the ability to restore lost memory and functions! One physician has received approval from the U.S. Food and Drug Administration to begin testing a form of gene therapy in humans with Alzheimer's. What this researcher did was to implant genetically modified cells that deliver human nerve growth factor (NGF) into the brains of monkeys that showed age-related declines due to atrophied brain cells. NGF is a substance that nourishes brain cells. In the tests, NGF revived degenerated brain cells linked to memory, selective attention and other key factors in the thinking process. Also, a newly discovered fact that is very much contrary to popular belief, is that new brain cells continue to develop throughout life.

With this new information and the continued work in research, a cure could be right around the corner. Unfortunately, human testing could take years as will the final approval to make public any findings and/or conclusions. Then it takes more time to get the drugs on the market. So even though this "corner" looks close, it may still be ten to fifteen years before anything is available to cure or even prevent this dreaded monster from taking over the lives of so many families.

In the meantime, it is a long and hard battle with the certain knowledge that you will never win. It is the longest walk you'll ever take and the loudest silent scream you will ever hear. Some people have referred to Alzheimer's as the "longest good-bye." I prefer to think of it as an exercise in life. An exercise that will teach you things that you never knew you could learn and an exercise that will let that "other side" of yourself emerge. It can only make you a better person.

Just hang on.

Chapter 17

" . . . the system will not tell you."

Health Care Reform

This is going to be a tough chapter for me to write without my emotions running rampant and my fanatical and sometimes hysterical attitudes taking over. As you read on, you will see why my blood is already beginning to boil and I would guess that you can probably hear my teeth grinding over the radio or the traffic. But bear with me, and I believe that by the end of this chapter I will have you right in my back pocket. My hope is that you will drag yourself out of my pocket, take heed, and participate in my endeavor and become part of the raging masses. It ain't gonna be pretty.

Currently, Alzheimer's afflicts about 4 million Americans, some 3 million of whom live at home and are cared for by the family. As the baby boomer generation approaches 65, nearly 7 million Americans are expected to be afflicted with Alzheimer's. That would push the number of home-cared individuals to around 6 million. That's the entire population of a major American city! That could also be the entire population of one of our great states!

So what are we saying here? We are saying that that is a hell of a lot of people who will be unable to function. Mainly people who have worked all their lives only to be swept under the rug by the one entity that they spent their lives supporting. Our government.

Now let me make one thing perfectly clear before I go on lest I am tagged as some sort of disloyal dissident. I love this country and believe this country to be not one of the finest, but the very finest country in the world. I have friends and relatives who return from their homeland countries after a visit and all say the same exact thing. There is no place like the United States.

I feel blessed and privileged to have been born here and to be able to live my life in the midst of such prosperity and opportunity. There is nothing like an American supermarket anywhere in the world and there is nothing like the American election process, the American Constitution and the Bill of Rights, and a good old-fashioned 4th of July. I still get teary-eyed when I hear the Star Spangled Banner at a baseball game when the crowd goes nuts with applause after it's over.

However, as wonderful as it is, as most things go, it has its flaws. Now this could open a real can of worms because everyone is probably starting to make their list. Another great thing about this country. You can criticize it until you're blue in the face and don't have to worry about someone coming to get you in the middle of the night. But let's be fair, folks. We know that everybody's got a beef about one thing or another, but I would suggest you go and write your own book and let me continue on with mine and the subject at hand.

I discussed earlier the pitfalls to watch out for when you might need to apply for financial assistance from Medicaid or Medicare. But my main message in this book is focused on caring for your loved ones in your home, as was stated earlier when I mentioned the 6 million folks who will be afflicted and will need to rely on their families for in-home care.

Keep in mind that our government, i.e., our senators and congressmen, are making progress in certain areas of our health care reform campaign. They are currently looking at the prescription drug issue, capping outpatient co-payments, tax relief for purchasers of long-term care insurance, etc. But we still have a long way to go.

I mentioned the over-the-top expenses for nursing home care. I also mentioned what it costs for in-home care. These dollar amounts, for both nursing home care and in-home assistance, are most disappointing and frustrating. But my anger explodes when I recognize the facts as they exist in the middle class families. For instance:

Both my parents worked their entire lives, going well past their retirement age. During those years, approximately 50 to 55 years each, they paid every tax levied on them by various governments from federal to state to village to county to sales to real estate to God knows what. They paid into their Social Security for the required time and amounts. And they paid these taxes willingly and timely as law-abiding Americans.

And yes, there are certain senior benefits that were allotted to them, but nothing hugely memorable. We chose in-home care for my Mother mainly because of the kind of personal and daily attention that we knew we could give her, but also knew that we were not of a financial status to be able to afford a nursing home to the tune of anywhere from $3,000 to $5,000 per month.

In-home care or custodial care is what seniors most frequently need, but even those costs can be astronomical to the average working class family. These costs can run upwards of $400 to $500 per week. Granted, at that rate, it is cheaper than a nursing home, but I don't know of many families who can even afford that, much less folks who may be on a fixed income. Something needs to be done.

But Congress has sent us a message. And that message comes in the form of the Health Insurance Portability and Accountability Act of 1996. This law provides tax incentives for the purchasers of long-term care insurance. In other words, the federal government is telling us loud and clear that it has no intention of funding any long term care program for our afflicted elderly.

I don't understand how our government can spend millions of dollars, or even billions, on things that make no sense. $60 million alone was spent on attempting to prosecute a president with an overactive libido. Who cares. I didn't. My family didn't. My friends didn't. And most Americans didn't. That $60 million would have afforded in-home care for 3,000 victims for an entire year.

We have 13 and 14 year olds getting pregnant and immediately going to the welfare system because they aren't old enough to get jobs. We have people coming into this country whose first lesson is how to get on the welfare system. We have women irresponsibly continuing to have children while on welfare and doing nothing about getting themselves off the system. I get a huge kick when I stand in line at the grocery store with my hamburger, hot dogs and canned spaghetti while a welfare recipient is in front of me buying steaks, roasts, and ribs with food stamps. Granted, there is a great number of people educating themselves and working diligently to get themselves off the system. Unfortunately there is a larger number doing nothing. And our government is doing nothing about them.

Yet our seniors, who have worked for 50 years and payed taxes all those years, can get no relief whatsoever when they become afflicted with a debilitating disease like Alzheimer's and desperately need help caring for their spouses, but can't afford to go elsewhere for that help. Something is out of balance and someone needs to stir up a little fire from the embers.

I have included on the following pages two letters. One to send to your State Senators and one to your Congressmen. We are always told that writing to your Senators and Congressman does make a difference. I would like to see just how much attention is paid to these letters that we are encouraged to write and what response, if any, we may receive. More importantly, what changes will be made.

When I listen to our politicians, I always get a laugh when I hear the phrase, "Well, the American people feel . . ." or "the American people say . . ." I don't ever remember any politician asking my opinion on any subject. Or any politician asking me what my needs are as an American citizen. Well, here is our chance to let them know just how we do feel on THIS subject. Subjects that matter and subjects that are pressing. As each day goes by, millions more become afflicted and millions of families embark on this treacherous journey of survival.

And know one thing. Currently, on the Internet, you can go into the U.S. Government web site and look up the voting record for each and every politician currently in office including what bills they have introduced to the Senate and Congress and exactly how they voted on each and every issue. This public voting record capability will give us the ammunition we need when it comes time to elect or re-elect any of our politicians. Watch it carefully.

Please participate in this endeavor and let's be a voice that can be heard for years to come. Because in years to come, we are going to need more help than ever.

I have included a generic address in Washington, D.C. for both Senators and Congressmen. You need to make an inquiry as to your specific state to get the names of your current Senators and Congressman so the letters can be addressed to your State's politicians. If you are so inclined, you can go ahead and send the letter directly to their State address. I have also included the address of the Senate Special Committee on Aging.

Office of Senator _____
United States Senate
Washington, D.C. 20510

Office of Congressman _____
United States House of Representatives
Washington, D.C. 20515

Senate Special Committee on Aging
United States Senate
Washington, D.C. 20510

Dear Senator _____ :

  I am sending you this letter today to let you know that I am part of a growing national crisis. That crisis is the ever-increasing numbers of afflicted individuals with Alzheimer's. Most of the population out here has or will have some connection somewhere with an individual suffering from this disease. A good number of us are already dealing with this disease in one stage or another.

  The even larger crisis is how are we going to take care of these folks. With nursing home costs at an already astronomical level and in-home full-time care almost out of reach for most Americans, we will have no alternatives for caring for our loved ones and no financial relief or assistance for that care.

  We are looking to our elected officials in Congress to take heed and begin a campaign to introduce some type of long term custodial care as part of our Medicare program. As life-time tax payers, we need to be afforded first priority and not be turned away because we did what appears to be an incredibly stupid thing. We worked our lives away and paid taxes, only to be swept under the rug in <u>our</u> time of desperate need.

  We will be watching any and all bills that are being introduced and watching the voting records of those elected officials from our specific States.

  We look to you for assistance in this matter and will expect your record to show that you are, in fact, working towards a solution.

     Respectfully,

     _____

     _____

     _____

Dear Congressman _____:

   I am sending you this letter today to let you know that I am part of a growing national crisis. That crisis is the ever-increasing numbers of afflicted individuals with Alzheimer's. Most of the population out here has or will have some connection somewhere with an individual suffering from this disease. A good number of us are already dealing with this disease in one stage or another.

   The even larger crisis is how are we going to take care of these folks. With nursing home costs at an already astronomical level and in-home full-time care almost out of reach for most Americans, we will have no alternatives for caring for our loved ones and no financial relief or assistance for that care.

   We are looking to our elected officials in Congress to take heed and begin a campaign to introduce some type of long term custodial care as part of our Medicare program. As life-time tax payers, we need to be afforded first priority and not be turned away because we did what appears to be an incredibly stupid thing. We worked our lives away and paid taxes, only to be swept under the rug in our time of desperate need.

   We will be watching any and all bills that are being introduced and watching the voting records of those elected officials from our specific States.

   We look to you for assistance in this matter and will expect your record to show that you are, in fact, working towards a solution.

   Respectfully,

_____

_____

_____

Chapter 18

" . . . from whole to half to zero."

Let The Rest of the World Go By

From here on in, it's up to you to take heed and begin your journey with the knowledge that I have attempted to transfer to you. It is your time to step up to the plate and take your position. To grab that sword and march forward with every inch of guts and determination you've got and with every ounce of knowledge you have learned. We've done the beginning and the middle. We've done the stories. We've done the informative and the humorous. We've made the lists. We've read all the instructions. We've been told about all the tips and signals.

Now I'd like to bring you up to date and into my home. My Mother, Alice, sits in her chair and stares into nothingness. There are days where she catches a tiny, tiny glimpse of something remembered. There are days when her attention can focus, if only momentarily, on just one little thing. A television cartoon, a song, a bird outside her window. Anything and everything is her grasp to reality. Just a second of a breeze can stir her brain and put the tiniest of glimmer in her eye.

But my hand on hers, or my lips on her cheek are the things that help her frail and terror-ridden little body relax and bring her clouded eyes into focus. She, as I, relish those moments we spend together to just be Mother and daughter. I always have to tell her my name, but then she quickly remembers me and recognition shines in her eyes. She reaches for my arm to clutch onto, as though she will never let me go. I move closer to her and put my arms around her. I hear her muffled groan of joy and comfort when I squeeze her and spill over with love and longing to have just a few words with her. We sit motionless and speechless, our memories entwining around each other as tears begin to form. She reaches up to stroke my face or to button a button on my blouse like she did when I was a little girl. Her "mother" spirit still lives on and she is still "caring" for me as though she is sending me off to school in the morning.

I remember the shopping excursions and lunches. I remember late night television movies with popcorn, and morning coffee that would last for hours. I remember three-hour telephone conversations and the excitement of a forthcoming week-end visit from her. I remember butterflies in my stomach when I was waiting at the train station as her train pulled in, inch by inch. All a distant memory and a painful realization that the only thing permanent in life is change. When they tell you that life can throw you a curve, they don't tell you that just around that curve is a brick wall waiting for you to slam into it. And by the time you get to it, it's too late. Too late to go back. Too late to change anything. Too late to redo those things you wish you could undo, or those things you wish you had done. The only thing left for you is to go forward and try to pull all the loose ends together.

Honor the spirit that you see before you. Remember the afflicted loved one with all the joy that was once there. And bring every ounce of love that you can muster up and let it glow all around. They will feel and respond, if only slightly, and it will make a huge difference in their existence, as meager as it will become. It is your job as a human being to care. It is your job as a human being to love. You've got tons of it in there. Perhaps your life situation, or your rotten childhood, or whatever your excuse might be, will be your reason for not letting it come out and be noticed. Trust me, you will do so much for your loved one and surprise! You will do so much for yourself, once it starts to flow, you won't be able to shut it off. You will ache so hard with love that sometimes you're going to feel like an explosion waiting to happen. You will sit at your job and suddenly be so overcome with a yearning to be with your loved one, you'll almost walk out the door. Love is magical and mysterious. But love is the only thing in this world that continues to exist without predisposition or reconstruction or re-learning. It is just THERE and will always continue to be THERE, no matter how hard you try to fight it or change it or ignore it. The easiest and smartest thing to do is to just GO WITH IT!

For our loved ones, you have to create a comfort zone. A place they can rely on to always be there. That place is your love. Imagine yourself with amnesia. Your first emotion would be fear. But if there were someone close by to take your hand and tell you everything will be alright, your fear and anxiety would diminish. So it is with Alzheimer's victims. Love IS the answer. I watched, daily, as she went from whole, to half, and now, nearly zero. Every day I poured out whatever I had to give and she sucked it all up. Clinging, grasping and searching. But she knew it was there because she knew I was there. She is still my darling and will always be the strength of my life, but, today, I walk with heavy heart and always on the verge of a desperate cry. The one thing that saves me from completely losing control, not for myself, but for her, is that she lived a good life with a daughter that adored her and a husband that worshipped her. He was an "old school fart" and could be the biggest curmudgeon going, but yet, he put my Mother on a pedestal and no matter what, she was his shining star.

My Mother and Father had a song that was "their song" for many, many years. They would get on stage at sing-alongs and sing it together, hand in hand, looking into each other's eyes, filled with love and admiration. Today, I still sing it to my Mother and when she hears it, her body straightens and she looks right into my eyes. She remembers her "pal," my Dad, and tries very hard to sing the song with me, but has a hard time remembering or forming the words. The song is very, very old and goes like this:

> With someone like you,
>> A pal so good and true,
> I'd like to leave it all behind,
>> And go and find

> Some place that's known,
>> To God alone,
> Just a spot,
>> To call our own.

> We'll find perfect peace
>> Where joys will never cease
> Out there,
>> Beneath a kindly sky.

> We'll build a sweet little nest,
>> Somewhere out in the West
> And let the rest
>> Of the world go by.

She hasn't found her peace yet, and the world is slipping by although she doesn't know it. Her joys are few. My prayer is that soon she finds where her "pal" waits, the one who left it all behind, to go and find, that place that's known, to God alone. I know there's a little stage up there with a little band just waiting for them to make another "appearance."

In the meantime, I still do what I can do. I kiss and I hug. I stroke her withered little hands and kiss her dried lips, brush her hair away from her pained face and wondering eyes. I pour love until my throat closes and my heart aches, continuing to smile all the way to let her know that "everything is okay." I watch her fade and wither, daily, slowly approaching zero.

She taught me love. I want her to know that what she taught me meant something. So I will be there when her eyes close for the last time so she can see the love and devotion that I have for her after years of giving of herself for me. I will be there to hold her when I hear the last gasp of breath. I will be there to fold the blanket one last time over her feeble little fingers. That's my job. That's <u>our</u> job.

It's the least we can do . . .

. . . for our Fading Angels.

Epilogue

I am told that this is not the end of my story, that I am not finished with this disease and that there is more to come. I am told that I still have decisions to make and that I need to convey more information to the public on the end of this disease.

My decisions have been made. That was part of our pre-planning many years ago.

Currently, I choose to live day to day and will face whatever comes when it comes. As of this printing, my Mother is still alive and a part of my life. As far as conveying further information on the end of this disease, I cannot write about what I do not know. But I do know the "end" of this disease hovers over me daily and I stand as tall as I can in the face of it. My hope is that, somehow, my Mother knows I'm here.